M000034623

The Ayurvedic Lens

Magnifying the Mysteries & Abundance of Life

A practical guide to healthy living
in a complex world

Dr. Meghana Thanki, NMD

Dr. Meghana Thanki, NMD Books are available for order through
Ingram Press Catalogues

This book contains information to be used as general advice on
health care. It is not intended to be a substitute for the medical advice of a licensed physician. The reader should consult with their
health-care provider in matters relating to his/her health and particularly with respect to any symptoms that may require diagnosis
or medical attention prior to making or implementing any changes
based on this book.

Dr. Meghana Thanki, NMD
Visit my website www.ayurzona.com & www.secondnatureclinic.com

7140 East 1st Avenue, Scottsdale, AZ 85251

Printed in the United States of America
First Printing: January 2017
Published by Sojourn Publishing, LLC

ISBN 978-1-62747-175-6
Ebook ISBN: 978-1-62747-176-3

Lord Dhanvantari Prayer

श्री:

॥ धन्वन्तरिस्तोत्रम् ॥

ॐ शङ्खं चक्रं जलौकां दधदमृतघटं चारुदोर्भिश्चतुर्भिः
सूक्ष्मस्वच्छातिहृद्यांशुक परिविलसन्मौलिमंभोजनेत्रम्।
कालाम्भोदोज्ज्वलाङ्गं कटितटविलसच्चारुपीतांबराढ्यम्
वन्दे धन्वंतरिं तं निखिलगदवनप्रौढ़दावाग्निलीलम्॥

॥ इति धन्वन्तरिस्तोत्रम् संपर्णम् ॥

om shankham chakram jalaukam

dadhad amruta ghatam charu dorbhi chaturbhih

sukshma svacch ati hridyam sukha pari vilasanam

maulim ambhoja netram

kalam bhodojo valangam kati tata vilasan

charu pitam baradhyam

vande dhanvantarim tam nikhila gada vanam

praudha davagni leelam

I bow to *Lord Dhanvantari*, who in his four beautiful hands is holding a conch shell, a disc-like weapon, a leech, and a pot of heavenly nectar. Through his heart and around his head shines the most pure and gentle beautiful blaze of light, also emanating from his lotus eyes. On the dark blue water his body is luminous, splendid, and shining. His waist and thighs are covered in bright yellow clothes. By his mere play he destroys all disease like a mighty forest fire.

Excerpt from Ashtanga Hridayam by Vaghbhata

Chapter 1: Ayushkameeya Adhyaya
"Desire for a long life"

रागादिरोगान् सततानुषक्तानशेषकायप्रसृतानशेषान् ।
औत्सुक्यमोहारतिदाञ्जघान योऽपूर्ववैद्याय नमोऽस्तु तस्मै ॥

ragadi rogan satatanusaktan asesa kaya prasrutanasesan

autsukya moharatitan jaghana yo purva vyidyaya namosutu tasmi

Salutation to *The Unique and Rare Physician*, who has destroyed, without any residue all the diseases like *Raga* (lust, anger, greed, arrogance, jealousy, selfishness, ego), which are constantly associated with the body, which is spread all over the body, giving rise to disease, delusion, and restlessness.

Acknowledgements

I extend my deepest gratitude to the healing art of *Ayurveda* and the countless ways in which it has enriched my life, my craft, and my journey. I give thanks to those beings whom inspired and informed my work as a physician. I owe the greatest of life's honors to my parents (Luna Viva Ananda and Mahendra Mehta) and grandparents (Drs. Kamala and Bhogilal Gandhi), who are also physicians, my husband Yagnesh for his unquestionable support, my two sisters Pooja and Meera for their tenderness and love, my uncle Dushyant Gandhi for his clarity and strength, and my daughter Veda for all she has taught me about myself. I thank my gurus and teachers whom faithfully shepherded me along the path of *Ayurveda*, beginning with Dr. Paul Dugliss, Dr. Suhas G. Kshirsagar, Vaidya Yashashree Mannur, Vaidya Dilip P. Gadgil, Vaidya Vedhas Kolhatkar, Vaidya Rasik Pawaskar, and Jonny Kest. I give thanks to Tom Bird for his guidance in writing this book and in helping me access my authentic self. Finally, I thank all of the patients whose lives I have had the privilege of touching and those whose lives I have yet to touch. I shall remain forever humbled and inspired by you all.

Contents

Foreword

by Dr. Suhas G. Kshirsagar BAMS, MD (Ayurveda)

The Ayurvedic Lens is a wonderful book written by my dear friend and colleague Dr. Meghana Thanki. This is an excellent guidebook for Mindful living. She has intricately woven her own life journey with a complete understanding of "true natural medicine."

Ayurveda, as we translate, is the science of life. We must understand the impact of life experiences on both health and disease. The rich tradition of *Ayurvedic* medicine dates back thousands of years, and now modern medical research is finally catching up with the vast and vibrant understanding of its medical philosophy.

Meghana is a wonderful soul who I've known for the last 10 years and I have witnessed first-hand her journey in the medical field. I have always admired her devotion, clarity, and the ease with which she distills the most complex Vedic principles into simple steps of Mindful Living.

The Ayurvedic Lens is like a prism that disperses the visible white light into a spectrum of life's most vibrant colors. The very basis of Ayurveda is to enjoy life and expand happiness. We need to be self-referral about who we are and the choices that we make in order to be healthy and happy.

The latest science of Epigenetics, Nutrigenomics, and Personalized Medicine clearly validates the *Ayurvedic* Dosha theory of Mind-Body Types and the importance of daily and seasonal routines. The latest science of Chronobiology tells us to respect the laws of nature. We need to follow the rhythms of nature to regulate the clock genes and avoid the onslaught of chronic disease.

The new advances of Genomics make it very clear that one's genes express whatever one desires. Genes can be turned on and off with thoughts, feelings, and emotions. This is precisely why *Ayurveda* is a true science of life. We believe that health is a byproduct of enlightenment. You need to be spiritually evolved to deal with the polarities of mind and body. The mind-body system is like a feedback loop where your self-care or self-neglect will affect your lifestyle, inner and outer environment, behavior, past conditioning, and beliefs.

The Ayurvedic Lens is an inspirational journey that clearly highlights the importance of the *Ayurvedic* way of life in the quickly changing landscape of medicine around the world.

Once again, I welcome you on the wonderful journey with Dr. Meghana Thanki exploring *Ayurveda*. She has a unique way of translating ancient wisdom for a modern audience. She lives an *Ayurvedic* lifestyle and shows her readers how to apply these practical principles to their daily living. *The Ayurvedic Lens* is a great start for you to find your own path to Health and Wholeness.

Author of: *The Hot Belly Diet*
www.AyurvedicHealing.net

Introduction

We all have a desire to heal. We also have a deeper desire to embrace the journey into healing. Some wait until a disease completely takes over, some wait until the onset of a few symptoms, while others, who are fortunate enough to have the right knowledge and tools, don't have to wait at all, thereby preventing the onset of disease before it ever begins. Why did I use the term *to heal*? Because *to heal* is a verb, and verbs necessitate *action*. *To heal*, by definition, is *to become healthy or well again; to restore to health*. To restore and maintain that balance is a constant process that takes repeated effort, time, energy, and dedication. And, why choose the word *desire*? Because *desire* is a *strong feeling of wanting or wishing for something to happen*. I believe most of us are still in this mindset. We desire for positive outcomes, but our own resistance (and even unknown resistance) to the effort it takes creates a barrier. Change is hard work and takes discipline, consistency, and commitment. Our dietary and lifestyle choices are driven by powerful conditioning, which can be largely unconscious, leading to disease.

We are all faced with many responsibilities in life such as career, building a family, maintaining the home, and keeping our relationships kindled. There is so much to do and so little time. The last thing we have time for is ourselves. There are too many convenient excuses. Unfortunately, for most people, worrying about health comes last. Western medicine has trained us to only seek help when symptoms set in or when a set of symptoms creates disease. Preventing disease has not been ingrained in our cellular intelligence as something we should also have at the top of our list.

The health system in America has helped shape our ideas. Most of us have an annual physical exam, but that is rarely enough to motivate us to play an active role in our own health. That exam doesn't teach us to take responsibility for our own well-being; it's more of a green or red signal. We really should want to be living in a state of constant yellow—proceeding with caution, watching each thought, each action, each feeling, and each piece of food we consume. Everything we partake of should be met with a certain amount of awareness, striving to be present in each moment rather than sitting back and allowing disease to catch up with us.

In order for this to happen, we need to keep our health at the forefront of our thoughts. In doing so, we will see the other areas of life naturally leveling out. *Why?* Because we are living in tune with nature. Living against nature's rhythms disconnects us from our own biorhythms. These biorhythms are essential to recognize. Aligning ourselves with nature connects us deeply to our health needs... our inner wisdom.

What do I mean? For instance, take the experience of enduring an all-nighter. Whether frequent or rare, take note of the body's response. How do you feel the next day? Nature purposely retreats at night for us to rejuvenate and feel rested when we awake with the sun's energy. If we don't get the rest we need, it seeps into the rest of our day. We often find ourselves feeling groggy upon awakening, perhaps reaching for umpteen cups of coffee to get through the day. We might become irritable and our relationships with our loved ones begin to suffer, which ultimately leaves us feeling stressed out and depleted. We come to find out that it was a waste of time from the beginning. In this way, these simple daily rhythms become indispensable to our well-being.

The next question arises. *How do we know what is right and what is wrong?* There are so many fads out there. We all get bombarded with the latest and the greatest—the juices, the fasts, the exercise routines, the diet plans, weight loss programs, and new supplements. My best attempt at answering this question comes down to understanding your body and not blindly following any one of these, rather following it because it makes sense to you and your body. You will know if it feels good if you pay attention. We have to become our body's best observer. We are only going to stick with something if it makes sense and makes us feel good. Therefore, my advice to you is not to do what others feel is right for you. If you feel eating a warm, cooked meal is leaving you less bloated and gassy consistently then you are on the right track. If you feel getting to bed on time and waking on time leaves you rejuvenated, then you are also on the right track. It is important to note that the simplest changes in diet and lifestyle can shift your health dramatically.

Now that we have a parameter to judge whichever system of healing we choose, I'd like to introduce to you the oldest system of healing known as *Ayurveda*. *Ayur* means life and *Veda* means science, which translates into *the science of life*.

We are in fact talking about the art and science of life. They are interwoven; they are two sides of the same coin. Science is logical, pragmatic, and left-brained while art is right-brained, creative, and imaginative. Mixing the two, we have a method to take care of the body, mind, and spirit, moment by moment, day after day.

Science has always intrigued me. *Where does energy come from?* I wondered this as a young girl. Why didn't we have to plug ourselves into the wall in order to function? From where did this seemingly infinite supply of energy come? I loved learning about the human body, which led me to taking science into my own hands by majoring in chemistry and completing my naturopathic doctorate, eventually diving into the deep, vast ocean of the science of *Ayurvedic* medicine.

Retrospectively, I recognize that my curiosity about life has led me to make a deep connection between the visible and invisible. I was passionate about uncovering the mysteries of my relationship with myself and others. The tools I have gathered on my journey have certainly cleared my queries and allowed me to hover in the glow of the yellow light where I continue to heal.

How will reading this book benefit you? If you open yourself to its message and choose to *act*, you will become inspired to take your health into your own hands. You will begin to understand that the principles in this book are not meant to be blindly followed. You are meant to follow them when you discover that they aid in the true healing of your being. After all, our health is in our own hands and we are responsible for our own well-being.

You will gain great clarity into the mysteries of your life. It all started 5000 years ago with various forms of healing: Chinese, *Ayurveda*, Tibetan, and Greek. We then moved into a more western-oriented approach to medicine, marked by viruses, bacteria, technology, vaccinations, and pharmaceutical drugs. However, we are returning to these ancient methods of healing related to food choices, lifestyle, meditation, and yoga. We have come full circle. We have embraced the idea that our solutions lie within, using simple and accessible practices involving the mind, body, and spirit.

You will slow down the aging process from the inside out, and learn daily what to do rather than only when you are sick.

You will begin to discover your body. You will gain insight related to why you act and behave the way you do. You will discover what tips the scale and what brings you off balance. You will become your body's own best scientist. You will begin to answer your own questions about what to eat, how to eat, and what exercises are best for your body type. The different ways of viewing health and the world will become apparent as you fall in love with your being.

What else am I going to get? You may be asking this question. You are not going to get a magic pill that takes it all away—the pain and the suffering. However, you will develop tools that will help you on your journey. Practical, common, everyday tools that you won't blindly follow, but that make sense and create a difference. As you delve deeper into this book you will discover a path—a path that you can come right back to in case you lose your way.

Your body will work smarter, not harder. Your toxic load will decrease so that your body can function more efficiently.

You will discover that there is a roadmap for success at each stage of life: birth, youth, middle age, and old age. Sometimes the solution is simple and sometimes it is more complex. Either way, commitment to the process is essential.

You will enter into a creative journey with yourself using the science of *Ayurveda* as your guide. This ancient wisdom is awaiting your presence, as it will stand by you from the toughest of times to the happiest of times, and everything in between as you peer through an *Ayurvedic Lens*, journeying into your desire to heal.

CHAPTER ONE

Divine Light Rushes In

I feel the warmth of my daughter's hug and her soft hands as she strokes my face, indicating *Mommy it's okay. I'll be okay.* I can feel my heart beating with excitement and my eyes slightly heavy as they flood with tears. *I'll be okay mom,* she whispers once again. I couldn't understand. Was I happy, sad, or a bit of both? *I love you dearly.* I say this out loud. I must have repeated it 10 times before leaving. I had cried earlier that day as she lay in her favorite position across my chest, heart-to-heart, with her legs straddled to either side, falling asleep to the motion of the rocking chair. It was the first time since her birth that we were to be without each other. *What is going to come of today?* I whispered in her ear just as she was falling asleep. I am going to write about you, my dear. Oh, how we love each other! So unconditionally. It's now dawning on me that we have always been connected, and we will continue to be, no matter what comes our way. I feel you are *a part* of me. I watch so patiently to see what each day brings. You are a miracle, a true gift to your dad and me. I observe how you greet me, how you touch my face with those tiny hands, and how you just know. The tears have settled. I guess this is how the two of us will connect. I'll miss you these few days while I take time to write this book, but I know your divine light is rushing right through me. Your message to me is: *mommy you can do it. I believe in you.* I am so proud to be the mom of this beautiful, wise girl.

Her name is Veda. The *Vedas* are large, ancient texts written in Sanskrit originating in India. Her name translates to *knowledge and wisdom* and is derived from the root *vid—to know.* She is 14 months old (at the time of writing this book) and at the peak of exploring her *kapha* voice as she repeats *mama.* She reminds me daily of how all of our lives began. She's so uninhibited, and it's never more apparent than when she dances. Have you ever observed the layers of movement that unravel as a baby begins to dance? It starts as a simple bounce and a slight bend in her knees before it moves into a side-to-side motion of her hips. This is followed by a series of pelvic thrusts while she nods her head to keep the beat. What a delight! As soon as any music begins playing her routine is in full motion. She is a true representation of freedom. We all started this way until the protective layers around our authenticity began to restrict us, blocking our vision of life. She is a daily inspiration, with threads of pure love, joy, wisdom, and laughter running through her being and flowing into all those who surround her.

Her divine light rushes through with a message, reminding us of the beauty of life, how we present to the world, and those things that pull us away from our true being.

The memory of one of Veda's first words is so vivid. She looks up to the light, points, and repeats *ight, light.*

The Birth

The birth of this book, the birth of my daughter, the birth of myself, the birth of my marriage, and the birth of my practice. We are surrounded by birth. Everything in nature must be birthed—plants, animals, people, books, and even ideas. For example, the idea for this book was born from a brief conversation that I had with my mother during which I came to the realization that if I could give birth to Veda, I am sure I can give birth to a book that describes my journey.

It was five days before her due date, on Monday, September 16th, at about 3 am. We were in Old Town Scottsdale, Arizona, and the contractions had begun. I immediately alerted my midwife and doula. I had been sleeping in the guest bedroom because the height of the bed made it easier to navigate. I made it through the night, and eventually Tuesday morning rolled around. My mom and I managed to get out of the house to grab lunch and some groceries for the days ahead. In birthing terms, it's called a vacation day. We ate at an Indian restaurant nearby. The contractions were occurring every 30 minutes and very tolerable. We went to a local supermarket to pick up a few groceries, consisting mostly of items we were told to gather prior to the birth—honey sticks, popsicles, and coconut water, all of which proved indispensable later.

That evening my mom and I went for a brisk walk outside our condo. It was the middle of September, so there was a slight chill in the air. I was feeling positive and following everything I learned from the classes I attended. Walking was supposed to help with the positioning of the baby and make for a smoother, less painful birth. I made it through the night, and my body was showing every indication that the birth was proceeding. The mucous plug released and the contractions continued at about 8 minutes apart. As Wednesday dawned, I was in and out of the bathtub, not entirely sure what was happening. I had attended two birthing classes. Who has time for that? Well, I did. My personality was such that I had to be prepared. I joined one birthing class that followed *The Bradley Method*, also referred to as "husband-coached childbirth," which focuses on birth as a natural process. *The Bradley Method* espouses careful guidelines for prenatal diet and exercise, as well as tips for better managing labor with deep breathing techniques and the support of a labor coach. I also joined Pam England's *Birthing from Within* course, which offered guidance based on helping me discover my strengths and needs for a smoother birth. My husband and I were artists at work through the *Birthing From Within* class. I worked on uncovering what the birth might be like by facing my personal fears, doing *labyrinth work*, and listening to personal stories of other mothers who've become birth warriors. My husband participated in all of the activities. In one activity, he placed his hands in ice to experience what a contraction might be like and began to learn how to dig deep within himself to best understand how to support me. Each piece of artwork we created in class was taped on the wall in our living room so that I could draw on them for inspiration when the birth was tough.

It was now Wednesday evening. I kept calling my midwife. The conversations always revolved around the length of time between contractions. She was so confident in her birthing knowledge that she encouraged me to carry on with my daily activities and instructed me to call her back when the contractions were 3-4 minutes apart and I could no longer hold a conversation. "How does she know I'm not further into this?" I thought to myself. I remember feeling so frustrated. If only she could just come, put her hands on my belly, and assess my situation. I had my Bradley book open to the two-fold page titled "Overview of Labor and Birth," which listed the stages of birth in a table. I was trying to follow it like a textbook and I found myself repeatedly trying to determine which box I most belonged to: early first stage, late first stage, second stage, and so on. The length of the page filled with emotional cues, descriptions of contractions, and helpful reminders, specific to each stage of labor. This is not how I expected the birth to go.

I was also in touch with my doula, Pam. In hindsight, she was the most amazing person I could have asked for during the birth. She arrived on Wednesday evening while I was in the tub. Things seemed to progress when I was in the bathtub, but as soon as she arrived everything stalled. The contractions were faint and growing further and further apart. I made my way into the blue, blow-up birthing tub that was in the living room. Pam was guiding me through. As things seemed to slow down, I got out. My youngest sister Meera arrived around this time. She had flown in from New York. We had been talking about this day forever. At the time, she was a third-year medical school student and was anticipating her role in this birth. I knew deep inside that Veda must have been waiting for her. Being at the birth meant the world to Meera. She knew she wanted to be a part of it. And truthfully, I needed her.

Everyone started to wonder what was happening. Why the delay? Pam examined me a bit further and used her knowledge to help move things along. She had assessed that Veda wasn't positioned correctly. She had me wear a belt around my waist tied up with a piece of cloth to help tilt the pelvis and allow for correct alignment. I followed everything she said. It was this *pitta* part of me that was holding on. *Pitta* is an *Ayurvedic* term for fire energy. I could see that Thursday's Jupiter energy was in full swing as I watched that morning's sunrise after a rigorous all-nighter. My mom, my sisters Pooja and Meera, my husband Yagnesh, Pam, and I gathered on a couch in the living room for a pep talk, just as teams do before a game. I cried. I remember thinking: *What if this doesn't happen? What if I have to go to the hospital? What if, what if?* I felt completely hopeless, unsure of what was happening or where we were headed. Pam suggested that I have my prenatal chiropractor come to the house. She adjusted me as I lay on my turmeric colored couch, gazing up at the ceiling, hoping for some magic to intervene.

Later, I tried to get some rest, as part of me knew I would have to get ready for the night ahead. I cried in my husband's arms and sobbed on his chest, speechless. We both knew we had to stay strong and hold positive space for this little being to find her way. I wanted a natural birth. I wanted it so badly. In fact, looking back, I can now see that this was my breakthrough. All the birth stories in Ina May's book describe this tipping point. It was just what I needed. It was going to give me the drive to have this baby just how I had wanted. I had to let go of anything and everything I was holding onto. The universe heard me. Veda and I were aligned—a lesson in trust, patience, and the divine timing of the universe. In retrospect, even getting pregnant took time. I recall telling the doula that everything takes time. *Nothing worth having comes easily.*

By 2 pm on Thursday, September 19th, the contractions had picked up. It was 3-4 hours after I'd had my breakthrough. I made my way back to the red couch in the living room. We had the silly contraction timer on the iPad going. Of course, that was Yagnesh's idea. He was using it to time the contractions, which were now 7-8 minutes apart. The contractions grew progressively stronger, one on top of another. It was wave after wave of intense sensations as I lay on my left side. I could tell this baby was ready. Pam knew exactly where to place her hands as she pushed with her fists into my lower back, relieving my pain. As I am writing, I can't even describe the pain. The birth amazed me as I worked my way through the contractions with the help of my husband, doula, sisters, and mom, as they all took turns pushing into my lumbar spine. Time kept ticking.

I was back in the birthing tub in the living room by 6 pm. The crew had stepped out to get ice cream and dinner, leaving my husband and I alone. As we looked through the window, we could see the full harvest moon shining right into the room. It was a sight. My husband was leaning over the tub with his hands on my lower belly. He had this way of communicating with Veda. Not a day went by that he didn't kiss my belly and whisper, *I love you, Veda.* He didn't tell me, but I knew he was talking with her and telling her that this was going to happen. The contractions were becoming intense. It was 8 pm and my husband's intuition was at work. He called Connie, the midwife, and told her to come over and check me. The contractions were 3-4 minutes apart, and he could tell I was beginning to check out. Pam was also alerted. We spent a little more time alone in the tub.

The midwife, doula, and the midwife's assistant arrived at about 9 pm. The midwife proceeded to check me. By this time, the crew was back. Connie asked if I wanted to hear the good news. I said yes with all the enthusiasm I had after a fourth night of not sleeping. With a smile on her face, she told me I was 7 centimeters dilated and completely effaced. This baby was on her way out.

The midwife started setting up all of her medical equipment. She managed to cover our 8-foot long dining room table with all of her supplies. Let me take a minute to mention how amazed I was at her medical professionalism with regard to her attitude, her sterility, and her capacity to be equipped every step of the way. Meanwhile, I was roaming about the house as I still had three more centimeters to go. I was so happy. It was as if the midwife had finally given me the green light. She checked the baby's heartbeat. She was doing great.

It is funny what you recall looking back on those transformational moments in your life. It wasn't the waiting, the pain, or the discomfort. It was the long, blue, tie-dyed dress that was slightly crinkled and very bohemian in style that I remember. It belonged to my mom. She had several of those dresses in her closet and they were finally getting some use. I continued to walk around the house, swaying back and forth, holding Pam's hands as she cut my pain in half. She was magic.

Meanwhile, my mom was busy in the kitchen preparing an Indian sweet dish called *sheero* for use in an Indian prayer. In between contractions, I was actually helping her prepare the dish. I have pictures of this. Can you believe I was doing this? This wouldn't be possible in a hospital setting.

It was now about five hours prior to her birth. I was holding onto the granite countertop in my kitchen and inching my way across the house. As I was swaying on a birthing ball, I felt a gush of water, signaling that my water had broken. I was moving ahead. My baby and I were dancing. I got into the tub for a bit. There was a distinct feeling, as if my body was tearing apart. She was moving down. I felt my pelvic bones spreading and the warm water helped tremendously. Next came the hard part: the midwife checked me again and asked if I wanted to go ahead and do a manual cervical lip procedure. There was about 1 cm of dilation more to go. They never mentioned this in the birthing classes, but I trusted everyone at this point and did what they asked. I would say this was the toughest part. I lay on the floor near the tub, my mom and sisters at my head, and my husband to my right. The midwife successfully completed the procedure. It was a grueling 10 minutes. I just followed directions, screamed, and dug my heels into my husband's chest.

After being completely dilated, I began to feel the urge to push. I tried for a bit in the water. It was my dream for this baby to slide out into the water for my husband to catch her, just as we had seen in multiple birthing videos. After a while in the water, my midwife encouraged me to go ahead and get out. She was afraid I would become too tired and it would take longer. My husband prepared the other room, the one in which I'd been sleeping for the past few months. My family helped me make my way to a low futon, where I laid down. The instructions were to start pushing when a contraction came on. I remember some chaos around something to do with the internet connection and the midwife needing it for her data on her iPad. Believe it or not, I remember every moment of this process—true awareness. I pushed for roughly two hours. A funny moment occurred to me as Veda was starting to crown. Pam had been holding a mirror for me to watch Veda's arrival. I had somehow mistaken the top of her head for her nose and asked aloud if that was her nose. We were all laughing. This was happening. I pushed with all my might.

At this point, the doula and the midwife were both positioned at my feet, Yagnesh to my right, and Pooja, Meera, and my mom behind me. My mom and I locked eyes repeatedly. Somehow she gave me the strength I needed without saying a word. I remember telling my sister Pooja to come crouch behind me. I needed her there, holding my hand. Although we were in a tight space, my *pitta* nature dictated that I position everyone just right. I watched the whole process in a mirror the doula was holding. At the last minute, I even screamed for my husband to videotape the birth. We hadn't planned on it, but it all worked out. He made it happen, like always. In between the pushing, I was being fed pieces of this amazing strawberry popsicle. I would say this was one of the highlights of the birth. My sisters reassured me with their love while alternating cold towels on my forehead. My mom held space for me. Her hands were not physically on me, but whenever I looked up at her I could feel tremendous power and strength. It was so amazing. Her energy combined with the popsicle, cold towels, and my husband's hands were all I needed in that very moment. Veda was arriving at her own pace and rhythm. I had to be patient in the midst of angst and intensity. There was no definite answer to my persistent question *how much longer*?

Next thing we knew, my wise little angel was born. The time was 3:24 am early Friday morning. She didn't cry immediately. In fact, she didn't make a peep. It took a moment. She was placed in my arms, across my chest. I just laid there in awe. The first words out of my mouth sought confirmation, *it is a girl, right?* I was told many times, despite the ultrasound, that she would be a boy. We named this beauty Veda. She was born on a Friday, the day of Venus, three hours after her due date. My mom was amazed and told me later that she couldn't believe my strength. It was five days of what I now understand was a prodromal labor. I was so grateful to my family, the midwife and her assistant, the doula, my strength, the strength of the universe, and the strength of this miracle girl. I was in awe. She weighed 8 pounds, 1.5 ounces, and measured a tall 21 inches.

This process was extremely transformative. I birthed a baby naturally. My husband and my family witnessed this miracle, just as I had wanted. In the Bradley class, we read a book on husband-coached childbirth. Dr. Bradley used to tell dads that your child will say, "My daddy helped borned me."

What a moment of pride. I feel so fortunate that Yagnesh was able to be part of such a beautiful process. I was relying on him. We had practiced all the techniques together. He was the perfect labor coach for me. I used to imagine what it would be like, the birth. I was scared, but somehow I had faith. I was comforted, knowing that countless women before me had done this, and that I could too. The birth replays constantly in my mind. It reassures me of the power we have as women.

Through my preparation for Veda's birth, I had read every birth story in Ina May's book. I knew that one day I would write my daughter's birth story. Ina May Gaskin is a famous midwife in the United States. She oversees births in a village called The Farm, located in Southern Tennessee, near Summertown. She has put together a book of birth stories, as told by those who would travel from all over to birth naturally at her farm. The stories were incredible. They gave me inspiration and held me through until the end. Sometimes I would read them repeatedly. I was envisioning how my title would read: *Veda's birth—September 20th, 2013.* It is exciting to know that her birth story has found a home in this book.

Who is this lady that experienced this birth? My daughter reflects the answer in her most communicative of gazes. I felt her tender thoughts: *Mom, you are patient, loving, and caring. You are fully present. You massage me daily with warm oils and a loving touch. I think it's a game. I run and you drag me back. You are equanimous. You feed me with enthusiasm and birthed me naturally. You are the best mom, ever. You are a doctor, always giving me bitter herbs. No wonder I am an Ayurvedic child. You are a patient teacher, a loving wife, an amazing cook, a meditator, a guide, an inspiration, an Ayurvedic practitioner, and a beautiful woman, inside and out. I look to you as I absorb the world. A five-day birth process and the strength it took to get through breast-feeding—persevering despite all odds. I was present as you met with every lactation consultant possible. I commend you. A chemistry major and a panchakarma specialist, you have gone through all of this before me. You are qualified to teach the world how to live life with this recipe book for life, love, liberty, and laughter. I see your knowledge and your love for Ayurveda, so much so that you named me Veda.*

Who am I? I ask myself. I am someone who loves life, loves family, and loves to love. I am transparent and genuine—a true example of always being curious about my roots and the healing potential of the universe. *But why?* is my mantra. I am constantly trying to decipher and dig deeper. I work hard and remain dedicated toward my heartfelt goals.

My Journey into Medicine

My journey in preparing for the birth of my daughter started with the science of *Ayurveda*, a 5,000-year-old system of natural healing that has its origins in the Vedic culture of India.

My Indian roots are close to my heart. I started dancing from a young age, both classical Indian and folk. My relationships with my husband and family, along with my love for India, have conspired to bring me to this place of being. These experiences have held my hand on this journey and will continue to lead me, moment by moment, down this eternal path. Digging deep into the roots of my being has been the biggest gift I have given myself. It isn't surprising, given my grandfather's journey. My mom always told me he never stopped short until he found what he was looking for. He was on a quest, at one point, after having read the *Bhagavad Gita*. He was searching for a way to put those principles into action. He landed on *Vipassana* meditation, which will be discussed later.

My medical journey started the moment I chose to major in chemistry. I came to that decision after taking an organic chemistry class in college. I enjoyed studying the elements that make up our world. The periodic table became my bible, encompassing exactly what it meant to study chemistry. I had it memorized and color coded by the end of my school career. I had to be able to recall obscure facts about each element in my sleep.

Prior to modern chemistry, the ancient people had already developed a science by observing the five elements around us. These were ranked from least to most dense: air, space, fire, water, and earth. After observing these five elements in nature, they began to understand that the same elements also exist *within* not just *around* us. They understood that these five elements come together to form three *doshas* (or, the material substances in our body): *vata, pitta,* and *kapha.* These *doshas* have both a physiologic and a pathologic function.

What is My Message?

Who am I meant to touch through my writing? It's meant for those who feel burdened, stuck, or ill, and would like to clear their path. It is meant to help those who strive to feel lighter, happier, joyful... *more alive.* It's also for those who are tired of trying to figure it out on their own. It is a recipe book for living life in abundance. Does anyone have a recipe for success? I feel the desperation as I see the weary look in my patient's eyes. They seem defeated and lost, having tried many remedies. I can empathically resonate with the feeling. I hope to be a professional guide and educator. It's challenging, but rewarding.

This recipe book for life has a variety of ingredients: It's mainstay is *Ayurvedic* medicine with all of its lifestyle components i.e. meditation, cooking, oil massage, exercise, pre and post-partum care, detoxification, and journaling. This manuscript consists of the purest path in life I know of thus far. It will show you all the cards in the deck, the ace card being how to live a healthier, longer life. You will learn the best coping skills to help you through every stage of your life. It will help you dig into your roots, find out more about yourself, and explore your desires, your mysteries, and your story.

My hope is that you will not start all of this at once. The path begins with a single step. Being able to start at any point is the beauty of the system. My goal is for each of you to be able to observe the world through an *Ayurvedic Lens*, slowly incorporating the universal laws of nature into your being. Your curiosity will deepen as you gain an understanding of nature and the five elements.

Emotional, spiritual, physical, and environmental toxins surround us daily. It is up to us to know and feel what's right and what's wrong. *Ayurveda* teaches us how to tune into that. *Panchakarma* is a branch of *Ayurvedic* medicine specifically meant for detoxification of built-up *doshas*. These detoxification treatments allow our sticky, *dosha*-filled cabinets to empty, leaving us with a lighter body and clearer mind. *Vipassana* meditation, a non-sectarian technique, allows for eradication of mental impurities through self-observation. The 10 virtues of the *Buddha* begin to resonate throughout our being so that we may live a more peaceful harmonious life with both ourselves and others.

Slowly we must learn to relinquish living blindly and going through the motions. Our consciousness increases as we begin to incorporate different modalities. It is all there. And it is awaiting. Claim your potential. It is yours. The journey is hard and without end, but it is worth it. Evolve into your best person and cultivate your inner temple. We cannot be perfect, by any means, but we can know what tips us off and leads us away from peace. Remember the story about

Veda and her completely uninhibited dancing. When stressors build up in our bodies, we go into survival mode unconsciously. We tense and tighten up, clench our jaw, feel the weight of the world on our shoulders, shrink our energetic hearts, and become generally inhibited. Our goal is to get back to a pure, liberated space.

Each individual has a set of positive qualities that should be recognized. The key is knowing how these elements affect one's physiology and psychology, and ultimately, one's connection with others. For example, our fire could destroy us, or if well-kindled, promote growth. Our earth element could keep us apathetic and heavy or allow us to be dependable and solid. Our air element can make us flighty and erratic or allow for creative endeavors.

This brings us back to the understanding that we must heal ourselves in order to heal our relationships. Each one of us has significant relationships of varying responsibility and intensity. All of us have an innate desire to fulfill and live these relationships to the fullest. Wellness and ease are key ingredients to living gracefully in these relationships. It is my hope that this book will guide you on your path of wellness. It will offer a platform from which to understand the workings of the universe. You will begin to understand how we function, how we show up in the world, and what makes us tick. This book is a compilation of stories, patient cases, educational material, and an account of close personal relationships viewed through an *Ayurvedic Lens.*

CHAPTER TWO

The *Art & Science* Of Life

There are three great authors of *Ayurveda—Charaka, Sushruta,* and *Vaghbhata. Charaka* is the oldest and most important authority on the writings of *Ayurveda* dating back to 400-200 BCE. *Sushruta* is best known for his foundational work in surgery. *Vaghbhata* has written a set of books in a very poetic manner different from *Charaka* and *Sushruta.* The Sanskrit texts hold this powerful time-honored knowledge.

It is mythologically believed that the medical science of *Ayurveda* was handed down by *Lord Dhanvantari,* who was the personal physician to the Divine beings, for the benefit of those living on earth. He is depicted with four hands, each with a different tool. The first, *Shankh,* is a conch shell. It is believed that the vibrations which emanate upon blowing into the shell destroy disease causing germs in the atmosphere. The second tool being the *Sudarshan Chakra,* a mobile disc-like divine weapon with 108 edges. In his third hand are *Jalauka,* which are leeches used for bloodletting. Lastly, *Amrita* is a pot containing rejuvenating nectar. It is through *Lord Dhanvantari* that *Ayurveda* continues. Throughout all of my *panchakarma* treatments, I have and will continue to call upon him to offer his healing light and wisdom to both patients and myself.

Five Mahabutas

The *mahabutas* are depicted as the five elements that exist in nature from subtle to dense: space, air, fire, water, and earth. The ancients observed nature. They dug their feet into the earth, felt the warmth of the sun through its fire energy against their face, let the air battle against their skin, allowed various bodies of water to wash up against their entire being, and understood that anything not taken up by a material substance was space.

I recall my observations of nature and the five elements. I call it some of nature's best landscapes. It came to me that I must recap some of the most beautiful places I have been through an *Ayurvedic Lens.*

As I landed in the town of Cusco, Peru, I understood the air element at its best. I landed 10,000 feet above sea level. My breathing changed immediately, and I felt I was running after it even though it was there... silently working internally with determined focus. I managed to reach the hotel and sit down to eat, but during our practice hikes my situation became significantly worse. My breathing became shallow. A doctor came to my room to assess me. I was hooked up to a bit of oxygen and instantly felt relief. My *prana*, or life force, had been depleted. I had a perfect, real-life experience of a combination of *prana* and *vata* passing through my lungs. I was able to feel how my body reacted to such factors. Intimately. Nature revealed its power to me.

In Hawaii, we drove a distance at night and walked a long path up to an active volcano. I watched as the red-hot lava flowed down and fed the water below. A perfect depiction of the two elements, fire and water, that depict *pitta dosha*.

Multiple trips to India allowed me to experience the earth element through the density present in the ancient temples: Qutab Minar in Delhi, Khajuraho, Vrindavan and Mathura, where Krishna roamed, and Mt. Abu, a famous hill station. The intricate carvings were where ancient wisdom was hidden, depicting the solidity of the earth element and the beauty, softness, and knowledge that shines through, unspoken.

Picturesque moments still stand clear in my mind depicting the water element in its various forms: the beautiful Taj Lake Palace in Udaipur, the Argentinian Falls de Iguazu, prayers being performed with giant *divos* that spanned the Varanasi river banks of the Ganges, and the Niagara Falls, which I frequently visited as a kid.

Space is primarily depicted through sound. I immediately resonate with the vibrations that mantras carry with them. A specific moment comes to mind, when we approached the monastery at Bodh Gaya and the sound of Tibetan hymns were penetrating out into the entrance of the building.

Recall that there are five elements that come together to form the three *doshas: vata, pitta,* and *kapha. Doshas* are material substances in the body which have a specific, physiologic function. When they become vitiated through a variety of causative factors, most often related to diet and lifestyle, they become pathologic and take part in the formation of disease.

Vata is made mostly of air and space and is responsible for all movement in the body, from the gross movement of our limbs to the subtle movement of our blood flowing and nerves firing. *Pitta* is composed of fire and water and is responsible for transformation, not only with respect to our digestion but also as it pertains to the larger transformations that occur as we experience life. *Kapha* consists of earth and water and is responsible for the structure, strength, and immunity of our body.

It's imperative to understand the idea of *prakruti* (constitution) vs. *vikruti* (imbalance). With all of the information out there, it's easy to misunderstand this concept.

A key understanding in *Ayurveda* is that at the time of conception our constitution is determined. It can be a combination of the *doshas* above or just one. This doesn't change, and so allows us to understand that each one of us is unique and may react differently to the same situation. Understanding that our constitution doesn't change allows us to understand that *vikruti* is our changing condition. Our goal is to always return to our *prakruti*.

We begin to understand our inner workings as we watch the interaction of the various *mahabutas* (elements) within us.

Prakruti (constitution)

A balanced *vata* individual is usually depicted as having a tall, lean, physique. They tend to be artists, writers, dancers, and painters, using primarily their right brain.

My creative inspiration comes from my past, often through dance, beating my feet into the ground. My passion for the artistic nature of different dance forms allowed me to express myself and communicate. It is buried deep in my blood. I would compete in traditional Indian folk dance as a group. When we won, we would jump up and down with excitement, while losing would result in tears—we took it seriously. I also played a traditional instrument called the harmonium. I used to hit those keys with such rapidity with one hand as I would push on the accordion bellows with the other. *Ayurvedically*, these experiences can be interpreted as a way to channel *vata* energy into creativity.

A *pitta* dominant individual has a medium build and is very organized. For example, they may have their closet organized, not just into clothing types, but by color. Their car is clean. They have it all under control. They are loud and built to withstand. Digestion is fierce, as they are known to be able to digest just about anything.

My uncle took care of me as a young girl. He is an important person in my life. He is a true example of a *pitta prakruti*. Direct and accomplished, he has a golden heart that is soft on the inside and balanced by a hard outer layer. He is a true example of a leader, a strong personality who has journeyed through life and continues to make major shifts in his health and otherwise.

Kapha in balance is depicted by a person having a tremendous amount of physical and mental strength. The kind of handshake or hug they deliver can set this person apart. They are loveable, squeezable, huggable, rock-solid, dependable beings with an extraordinary compassionate space in their hearts to love others.

My husband is my rock-solid *kapha* guy. He has an immense capacity to listen. He contains an amazing soul I grew to love as I fell in love with my culture all over again—the language, the food, and the traditions. He grew up in India and spent the first 20 years of his life in a town called *Porbandar*, located in Western India along the Arabian Sea. He is a kind, caring, compassionate, loving, and giving man (not to mention, extremely handsome). He empowers me in the capacity to love as he does... unconditionally. He has given me our beautiful daughter, Veda. His *kapha* nature helps balance my *pitta*. He was very supportive during Veda's birth and lovingly participated in the birthing classes.

We see all types of individuals in the world, as we need them all. We need the *kapha* predominant individuals to serve the world with their compassion and the rock-solid strength they offer to a thriving business structure. The *pitta prakruti* individuals are needed for their capacity to stay organized and serve as leaders, and the *vata* type for a touch of the creative nature that the world needs to survive.

Vikruti (imbalance)

What is it that keeps us in balance? Our daily habits keep the *doshas* in balance through daily activities, including diet, exercise, sleep routines, attitude, and work. I imagine it as three separate jars: *vata, pitta,* and *kapha.* There are certain foods as well as lifestyle choices we engage in that begin to fill up the jars.

What is it that throws *vata* off? Lack of routine, thinking or worrying too much, intense activity (mental or physical), cold foods, ignoring our bodily urges, and any other lifestyle activities that add to the lightness, dryness, and mobility of *vata dosha.*

What irritates *pitta?* Spicy, sour, and fermented foods, anger, yogurt in the evening, excess tomato intake, alcohol (especially wine), and anything else hot, sharp, and oily in nature.

What weighs *kapha* down? Cheese, cold foods, ice cream, sugar, desserts, lack of activity, sleeping during the daytime, and any other causative factors that are cold and heavy in nature.

Previously, we discussed the understanding that *prakruti* is inherent within our being. We are now speaking of *vikruti*. What makes the *doshas vikrut*? Most of the *dosha* tests online help us determine our predominant *doshas*. What gets lost is the understanding of the difference between our core constitution and chronic imbalance. A common misconception is if we are predominantly *vata dosha* we only end up with a *vata* set of symptoms and, eventually, a *vata*-related disease. It might be more likely, but it is dependent strictly on our diet and lifestyle choices.

Therefore, even if someone has a *vata* constitution, he or she can end up with a complete *kapha* disease pattern. In other words, an individual can be thin and tall, appearing mostly *vata*, and have a consistent intake of cheese and heavy foods, which initiates a *kapha* disease process. On the contrary, a motorcyclist who has a *kapha prakruti*, but travels excessively daily in the open air can end up with a *vata* disease process. Yes, all it takes is one strong constant causative factor. The moral of the story is that when disease is absent then one can start paying attention to *prakruti* and bringing it into balance. But, once disease has started we must keep in mind the *doshas* that have accumulated or the tissues affected and then work backwards to unravel the disease process and begin healing. It is important to understand that these imbalances occur due to causative factors. It is not dependent on what *doshic* constitution reigns over us. It is when the *doshas* begin to collect that we see symptoms turn into disease. Each *dosha* has a set of causative factors that are responsible for creating imbalances in the body.

When a patient walks into the clinic without saying a word my work has begun. Dr. Rasik, one of my gurus, once explained, "My work is like that of a detective," referring repeatedly to Sherlock Holmes. I have now gained the skills to examine a patient by mere observation. I then begin to question which causative factors are at work. I inquire about exercise routines, food choices, emotions, traumas in life, bowel movements, and sleep, paying specific attention to how often certain harmful factors are repeated. I conclude with the use of an *Ayurvedic* hands-on exam, studying the tongue, pressing into the bone for tenderness and any signs of water retention, placing my fingers on the pulse, examining the muscle tissue, running my fingers across the nail bed, placing one hand on the top of the head, and pressing into the abdomen to get a feel for *dosha* accumulation.

After a brief explanation of *Ayurveda*, I immediately point out the need to avoid any causative factors that were found. I explain that if we don't, the *doshas* continue to accumulate and the load becomes increasingly heavy, showing up as weight gain, hormone fluctuations, or skin disruptions, to name a few. We lessen the *doshas* with the use of herbs and cleansing treatments.

What is it that is making us sick and out of balance? Our repetitive lifestyle, food patterns, and attitude is what ails us. We spend so much of our lives eating. It would follow logically that what we put in must agree with our system, otherwise we will feel its detrimental effects. Modern medicine has shaped our understanding around only looking at the effects of certain substances rather than focusing on the *gunas* (qualities) inherent in each substance, as *Ayurveda* does. Knowing these *gunas* is helpful, as we can understand the *doshas* that get affected. For instance, air, bike, and car travel can significantly aggravate *vata*.

Ayurveda teaches us to increase our awareness by observing nature and watching the times of the day, as the ancients did, in order to become the best observer within our temple. The *doshas* come together with our seven tissues to create disease. *Ayurvedic* diagnostic tools are used to understand *doshic* imbalance. *Ayurvedic* and western medical diagnosis differ in their interpretation of the origin of the disease process. Therefore, with my *Ayurvedic* and naturopathic medical training, I am able to use both modalities in a meaningful way.

CHAPTER THREE

Two Prakrutis Coming Together

My love story began when I was a teenager. I had grown up watching many Indian movies as well as epic mythological stories of the Hindu religion, like *Mahabharata* and *Ramayana*. I recall bike riding to the nearest Indian store to exchange one video cassette for another as we made our way through a 32-part series of both epic stories. Excitement revolved around continuing and not missing a moment. Some of the first few Bollywood movies I watched were *Saajan* and *Maine Pyar Kiya*. Very quickly, I began to idolize two Indian actors in those movies: Shah Rukh Khan and Salman Khan. What did these films have in common? Each had a central theme of love, just as in Hollywood. This shaped my image of whom I would marry.

Every woman has her dream man. In the late 80's, when I was growing up, it wasn't weird at all to put life-size pictures of Bollywood stars on your bedroom wall and I did just that. I had Shah Rukh Khan and Salman Khan greeting me daily as I walked into my bedroom. This set the stage. I knew that someday my Shah Rukh Khan would show up. I eventually learned that timing is everything.

At the age of seven, a nanny came to live with us and take care of us just as my youngest sister was born. We called her *Masi*, which translates into aunt. Her daughters came to live with us as well. Over the course of 10 years, our relationship with these girls became a close friendship and ultimately, we morphed into a family of five sisters. After they no longer lived with us, we were invited to Masi's oldest daughter's wedding. That's where Yagnesh and I locked eyes for the first time ever. Ironically, Yagnesh, who would become my husband, was also the nephew of my assumed aunt. He remembers having asked me for some french fries. Although, little more was said between us, he told me later that he knew immediately that I was the one. He was 20 years old at the time, having just moved from Porbandar, India, to the United States. He had been in America for only a year; he hardly knew any English. This poor guy, everyone doubted him: his mom, his aunt, his cousins, and so on. Yagnesh, being new to the United States, not having traversed the ropes of this land of opportunity, was advised to leave me alone. Everyone knew I came from an educated family. He did what he was told. He knew deep in his heart if we were meant to be together we would meet again.

And so our paths crossed once again at the youngest daughter's wedding. The irony is that he wasn't going to go to the wedding. It was being held in New York. I was not going to go either, but we talked it over as a family and we decided that we must go—she is like our sister after all. I had spoken with a dear friend before leaving and she mentioned to me with foreboding confidence: *You never know, weddings are a great place to meet people.* We ended up making the trip and there he was again, three years later. He was wearing a black and white suit as he made his way down a flight of stairs at a motel in Queens, New York. Our hearts started beating together. He looked familiar, and I heard myself say, *I've seen you before.*

During the rest of that weekend we kept connecting in various ways: sitting with each other during the ceremony, taking a trip outside in the snow to get some film for our cameras, venturing out to the flea market, and eating together. We rolled through all the mundane questions just to make sure we were headed down the right path. *Do you have a girlfriend? Where do you live? What do you do?* There was no girlfriend, he lived in Los Angeles, and he worked in the electronics industry. I was single, lived in Arizona, and was completing naturopathic school. The time we spent together was surreal. The wedding weekend ended as he dropped us off at the airport. He leaned over and whispered in my ear, "I am going to miss you." Was this magic or what? My Indian movie had begun. Our time together replayed in my head like a broken record. I still have the paper on which he wrote his name and address.

He didn't wait long to call me. Two weeks later, he made the drive from Los Angeles and we met up in Arizona. We went to Sedona together. Our time there resembled a scene from a Bollywood movie. We were lost in each other's arms with hardly any exchange of words, just feelings. I remember coming home after our trip to Sedona and picking up the phone to talk with my mom. I instinctively announced, *this is the guy.* My heart was singing. It was at this time that Yagnesh and I began to talk for hours about anything and everything. Of course, it was mostly on the phone. Gujarati, my native language, came alive. What a miracle. I had been spoken to in Gujarati and understood every word, but I became used to replying only in English. My mother and grandmother always spoke with us in this language and we would laugh, as some things are just funnier in your native tongue. This was a beautiful time. Shy at first, but I was encouraged word by word to speak Gujarati with him. And it was perfect, as it allowed me access to speak with his family.

Long distance was challenging. Our weekends were magical as we paid a visit to every beach in the Los Angeles area. Our love for each other grew and grew, just as the waves of the ocean build on top of one another. I learned so much about love from him. We laughed, but weren't entirely joking, when we referred to him as "the love guru." I was clueless, as I doubted our love at times. I kept feeling like the love we had was so strong while we were together, but then it would dissipate as we were apart. He once gave me an analogy that put everything into perspective. He said that the special love between us, buried deep in our hearts, was like searching for a particular garment at the bottom of a pile of laundry. He said the heart was the same. There are layers of the heart and our memories are buried inside. You have to uncover the memories and keep them close in order to keep the love alive. I found his words timely and profound. He taught me lessons in love. He was truly my Shah Rukh Khan. Funny enough, he even looks like him.

Eventually, we had to face some of the true questions of life, mostly related to where Yagnesh was headed with his career and where we would eventually settle down. I told him I wanted to stay in Arizona close to my family. After a lot of struggle, he realized his love for me was so strong that he would do whatever it takes, even if it meant moving to another state away from his family to be with me. Yagnesh stuck by me in the toughest of times. He cleared up my doubts and stood strong when I wavered. We made it, and continue to make it, through life's challenges.

One of the biggest challenges was when Yagnesh and I would part after a 3-day weekend in Los Angeles. It was a romantic love scene that replayed in my head. I would cry from the deepest place within. I've shed many tears saying goodbye to this man. I would get on the plane or drive back from Los Angeles and try to digest the weekend. I would arrive back to my home in Scottsdale, where my youngest sister and grandma were also living. My mom was also traveling back and forth from Michigan. We would have to part from her, too. *How could the heart hurt this much?* I would wonder. I have always been a soft, emotional being. Yagnesh, my sister, my mom, and I grew to dislike these sorrowful Sundays. It would take a day or so to recoup. It was during this time that I began to understand the capacity of the heart to hurt. In Sanskrit, the heart, or *hruday*, is the seat of *manas*, or, the mind. I had to pass through this. It was a test of the heart's capacity. According to *Charaka*, our entire waking consciousness rests in our heart.

Despite our conflicts, our hearts sang even louder. I had always wanted an Indian man in my life with the ability to create a relationship based on a love that keeps growing. We have a picture in our home that speaks to this. We were standing in front of the statue of liberty in Las Vegas. Here, we told each other that this was no ordinary path. This was a path that we were going to have to pave. Traditionally, an arranged marriage would have been in order for him, but we were perfect for each other. Our love grew leaps and bounds through the language, culture, family, and food we shared. In a nutshell, our Indian roots connected us.

After four years of long distance, having read every relevant long-distance relationship guide out there, it became clear to me that I would one day write my love story through an *Ayurvedic Lens*. In some ways it was love at first sight, while in other ways I had to grow to love him. *The biggest lesson in love was that it took time.* It takes time to get to know someone. I had to give permission to my heart space to fill with his love—that was the only way. I kept my memories and reasons for loving him close in mind until my heart knew. If I started using my mind, I would doubt it all.

My study of *Ayurveda* came at the right time. It gave me a lens through which to view and understand relationships. Through my own relationship as well as observing couples around me, I noticed expectations for one another kept surfacing. These expectations invariably lead to disappointment. Understanding our own *prakruti* as well as our partners was the only solution I saw to ease these expectations.

For instance, my husband's core *prakruti* speaks so truly. He is this bundle of love, compassion, and joy, always putting other's needs before his own, with emotional and physical fortitude. This is the true nature of *kapha*. I only understood I had chosen someone like this after studying *Ayurveda*. If ever I caught myself saying he didn't have certain qualities I was looking for, I simply had to remind myself of his *prakruti*. My nature reflects more of a *pitta* personality: analytical, organized, logical, sees things as they are, and in possession of a softness deep inside with a stubborn outer shell. This was the first time I was able to observe these *doshas* in another being and practice embracing my husband's *prakruti*.

Now, I see all beings like this. It's how I view the world. The key to marriage, relationships, and friendships is truly finding out what gifts the other person possesses and their core values and beliefs. We must work to keep these closely aligned. All three constitutions—*vata*, *pitta*, and *kapha* have their perks. Paying close attention and studying these combinations can help pave the way. This leads me to the understanding that we can't hope to feel complete through our partner alone. We must first do the work internally, in order to feel whole within. Being fragmented within only leads to a fragmented relationship with others. Understanding our *prakruti* helps us better appreciate the *doshic* differences in our partners. Only then can there be an understanding between two people. The foundation for a thriving relationship in my opinion is based on understanding *prakruti* as well as developing clear communication skills.

A specific discussion my sister and I had, prior to me getting married, comes to mind. It allowed me to gain clarity about my *prakruti*. The discussion was about whether Yagnesh and I should get married. We were driving and she asked me directly: *Meghana, what are you being so stubborn for?* It was in that moment I realized I was letting my head take over. My stubborn *pitta* nature was rearing its ugly head. It was up to me to make a decision. No one could do that for me. That moment stands in stark contrast to another memory of the surest I had ever been. My mom and I were sitting at a restaurant and I told her with all the confidence in my voice: *Mom, I love this man and I want to marry him.* Yes, there was my answer. It was out. The wavering was over. I had made a decision in line with my hearts desire. I was peaceful. I had stopped overthinking and tuned into my hearts vibration, very indicative of the inner softness of my *pitta prakruti*. To this day, I feel so happy about that decision. It was one of the toughest decisions I was ever going to make in life, one of such consequence and gravity, but I was certain that as long as we stuck by each other we could make anything happen.

My advice to couples now is at the end of the day, ask yourself: *What would make you happy?* For me, it is his stable *kaphic* nature as nightly he whispers *good night, sweet dreams, and sleep well*—never skipping a day. This is what I call love and deep commitment.

CHAPTER FOUR

The Three *Doshas*

Vata

Picture a tall, lean 33-year-old woman waiting at a bus stop. She has her earphones in as she listens to music on her iPhone, tapping her foot as a way to keep some sort of external rhythm. She searches through her bag, dropping several items on the ground before finally locating a tube of lip balm for her chapped lips. The bus arrives; she manages to find a seat and settle down. She nibbles on a few greens of a salad she had packed. A man occupies the vacant seat next to her and begins a conversation. She continues to jump from topic to topic, forgetting her stream of thought, demonstrating an extreme inability to concentrate.

Similarly, imagine a hyperactive 5-year-old child, who is running around the home completely distracted. He is unable to focus on much of anything including sitting still long enough to complete his meals at the table. These are examples of vata dosha out of balance.

Causative Factors

Vata is rampant in our society. We live in a *vata* toxic society worse than ever before. We are constantly multitasking, and as such are overwhelmed, tense, and stressed out. We are looking for a quick fix and much of the population begins to turn to mind-altering substances (like alcohol and drugs) when we should be seeking the exact opposite.

Vata dosha is responsible for 80% of all disease. It is good to imagine *vata dosha* as a marionette. We have to keep *vata* in control and manage it from above otherwise it loses direction and creates havoc.

One enters the *vata* stage of life after the age of 70, according to the Sanskrit texts. As we age, the oiliness starts to disappear from our tissues, our hair starts thinning, and our bones begin to crack. This teaches us to keep *vata* as balanced as possible through daily practices.

URGES

We have 13 different urges according to *Ayurveda:* passing gas, bowel movements, urination, thirst, hunger, sleep, coughing, crying, vomiting, sexual, yawning, burping, and sneezing. Consider a couple of typical scenarios we see today: *I will eat later, I don't have time before this important meeting or I had to stay up until 2 am, there was too much work to get done.* Our priorities are mixed up. These 13 urges are some of the greatest aggravators which set us up for a *vata* imbalance. If we skip bodily urges, such as not eating when hungry, not vomiting when nauseated, or not using the restroom when the urge is present, our *vata* gets aggravated. This is where awareness of our actions comes into play. Following these urges may seem simple, but ignoring them presents the likelihood of bigger problems down the road. Take, for example, the urge to cry. It is important to listen to this urge rather than suppress it. If a tragedy occurs, you must allow yourself to cry and process those emotions.

COLD FOODS

Raw food is becoming more and more popular these days. A key concept in *Ayurveda* is that food should be warm so that our *agni* (digestive fire) recognizes it as a like temperature. Raw, uncooked foods are cold in nature and over time will tax the digestive fire. The body will begin to slow down and not function optimally. We want to keep the *agni* stoked.

A very common question I may ask a patient pertains to *how* and *when* food is prepared. One out of every five patients will tell me how they, for example, prepare oatmeal for the entire week on Sunday, or how they will prepare soup and freeze it, then take it out as needed. What have we done? What have we become used to? These processes rob the life force: the *prana*, the *chi*, the *ojas* (vitality) from our bodies. We need to get into the habit of preparing fresh food daily and eating it the very same day while it is warm. Leftovers and frozen foods cannot give our bodies the proper nourishment or energy we require. It is little wonder the common complaints of low energy, constipation, sluggishness, and depression are saddening our culture.

COLD WATER

How many times have you gone out to eat and the first thing you are presented with is a big glass of ice-cold water, filled with more ice than water?

Now picture a small fire in the middle of your belly. What do you do when a fire is burning to keep it kindled? You add more wood. You don't add water. The same concept applies when we drink ice-cold water, as it puts out the fire we need to digest the wonderful meal that is about to be consumed. Therefore, the first thing we should ask for at any restaurant is room temperature water without ice. The water should be consumed during the meal, not before or after.

TRAVEL & EXERCISE

Excess travel is one of the most common ways to aggravate *vata dosha*. This is because when one travels one is in motion which is how *vata* accumulates. It can be from consistent travel in a car, on a bike, a plane or any mode of transportation. There was an example earlier of a man who rode his motorcycle daily for at least an hour. The open air brushing against his body as well as just being in motion created a *vata* imbalance. In fact, too much of any activity affects *vata*.

Many patients come to me with a history of running marathons. Excess *vata* begins to accumulate, and if not taken into consideration, a *vata*-related process will catch up with them. We must always be aware of the impact certain forms of exercise have on our *doshas*.

Misuse, disuse, or overuse form one key concept in *Ayurveda*. It teaches us that when we misuse or overuse one part of the body we end up creating a weakness where disease is likely to set in.

Yoga is one of the best forms of exercise to incorporate into our daily routine. It is the union between mind, body, breath, and movement. It is the sister science of *Ayurveda*. This focused breath allows us to increase the *prana* in the body. The backward and forward bending postures stretch the spinal column through its maximum range, giving a profound stretch to the whole body. I ask patients to perform 5-10 sun salutations after the application of oil. As the body heats up, the oil can penetrate deep within and lubricate our insides.

Exercise is important. When I ask about exercise routines, I find that oftentimes patients exercise in the evenings. Exercise is ideal between 6-10 am, when *kapha* is at its peak. Exercise must not be performed after eating because it can affect our digestion. According to the Sanskrit text, the person who partakes in daily exercise can brush away disease process. This is because the *doshas* are being digested through the *agni* created by the exercise itself.

ELECTRONICS

It has become common practice to plug ourselves into the TV, computer, or some other electronic device, especially in the evening hours. Doing so somehow gives us permission to become unplugged from ourselves. Cell phones have taken over our entire being as we are glued to them even when we are sitting with others. We have lost the ability to connect with those around us. We should start leaving all electronics aside after 6 pm, as we enter *kapha* time. During this 6-10 pm time, we should begin to calm our minds, unplug from our computer and electronics, eat dinner while carrying on meaningful conversation, and spend quality time with our children, our spouse, and our loved ones. It's important to realize this because we do the opposite. Picking up these habits will lessen the effect that *vata* has on our nervous system and allow us to settle down for a bedtime no later than 10 pm. If we go to sleep past 10 pm, *pitta* energy, what some call a "second wind," kicks in. *Pitta* time comes around again between 10 pm-2 am, and the body needs to detoxify during this time. If we are awake, the body's processes are disturbed. Getting into bed at the proper time allows us to both fall and stay asleep without the disturbance of our *vata* energy, permitting *pitta* to do its job.

How Do We Balance All of This?

Vata energy is present between 2 and 6, both am and pm. This is the best time for creative energy and grounding work like meditation and yoga. Our beings are the lightest as the sun is rising. We naturally should wake before 6 am. The body wants to get moving to dissipate the *kapha* energy that sets in. That is why if you wake after 6 am, or even more towards 8 am, you feel a heavier energy that makes it harder to get up and out of bed. The times of the day speak to us, and if we can follow them, we can live more in tune with nature and what it is asking of us.

MORNING ROUTINE

Ideally, we would each wake, take note of our surroundings, sit on the toilet in order to evacuate, brush our teeth, scrape our tongue, apply oil in order to perform a self-massage technique known as *abhyanga*, practice yoga *asana*, take a shower, eat a warm breakfast, and ultimately, start our day.

Abhyanga massage is a crucial part of the daily routine. *Vata* builds up cumulatively. Giving yourself warm oil massages on a daily basis helps pacify the *vata* that accumulates in our hectic lives. *Sneha*, which means love, is the Sanskrit word for oil, *ghee*, or any unctuous substance. Oil is our savior in *Ayurveda*. We use it because it is warm, unctuous, heavy, and grounding, the exact opposite of *vata*, which is cold, dry, light, and mobile.

Ayurveda works by using substances with opposite qualities to the *dosha* out of balance. *Abhyanga* pacifies *vata* immediately. The entire body can be massaged, from the toes up to the very top of the head. It is best to use round circles on round joints and long strokes on the long bones. The optimal oils for use in *abhyanga* are sesame, coconut, or a medicated oil. These should be warmed up before the massage. I recommend massaging yourself before exercising. This is because the heat produced from exercising allows the oil to penetrate inward, ensuring proper lubrication.

WHAT, WHERE, WHEN AND HOW TO EAT?

We should be eating in order to nourish the *dhatus*, our tissues. We have seven vital tissues that are nourished in *Ayurveda*: *Rasa* (plasma), *Rakta* (blood), *Mansa* (muscle), *Meda* (fat), *Asthi* (bone), *Majja* (bone marrow and nerve), and *Shukra* (reproductive fluid). The deepest essence of each *dhatu*, and the final byproduct of this entire way of nourishment, is *ojas* (our life force). We must be able to digest our food in order to enable proper tissue formation. There are visible signs of which to take note in order to determine the quality of each dhatu. There are also causative factors that can affect each dhatu, leading to weakness where *doshas* can accumulate.

I have been able to watch these *dhatus* build day by day. Veda to me is the depiction of someone with *dhatus* that are pure. Her daily foods (and mine) consist of mung dal, rice, ghee, milk, and wheat. As mothers, we are responsible for setting the stage for our children. We have control of what they are eating. As such, we should prepare the best food possible following the *Ayurvedic* guidelines.

I field questions consistently about wheat and milk allergies. *Ayurveda's* answer to this is that it comes back to digestion. Our *agni* is weakened, making it appear that we are allergic to these foods, when truly speaking, we shouldn't be allergic to anything. With the addition of spices and proper cooking combinations, we can avoid the allergic symptoms that some feel when consuming wheat and milk.

According to *Ayurveda* we should only eat when hungry and drink when thirsty. Another big misconception in modern medicine is that we are constantly told we must drink half our body weight in ounces. What a mistake. *Agni* has to digest the water that is consumed. Therefore, drinking only when thirsty is the rule in *Ayurveda*. Similarly, we don't just consume food because it is time to. We must listen to our hunger cues, being sure to eat when the body desires. When we do eat, we should do so while seated with as little distraction as possible. That means for example, we don't eat while standing, in the car, while multitasking, engaged in a heavy conversation, or while watching TV.

We should be consuming mostly home cooked food, where our love and energy go into the food and we have control over the ingredients used. We should be giving thanks to our food as we sit down, chewing mindfully, keeping one third of the stomach empty, and consuming room temperature water with our meals (rather than before or after). Lunch should be our heaviest meal, between the hours of

10-2 pm. This is *pitta* time, which means we have the sun to assist our digestive fire for optimal digestion.

THE FIVE MAGIC INGREDIENTS

According to *Ayurveda*, these five foods can and should be consumed on a daily basis for proper *dhatu* formation.

Milk—cooling, sweet, a warm drink at bedtime, nourishes *rasa dhatu*

Mung dal—easy to digest small, cylindrical beans used as an ingredient in soup, if too much ama has collected one can boil the beans in water and drink the water as a soup

Wheat—grounding, used for making chapattis (Indian tortillas)

Rice—grounding, nourishing, building

Ghee—nutty, aromatic, clarified butter, unctuous, rejuvenating, can apply on the bottom of the feet to cool the body down, great for the eyes and oleating your insides, can use to top oatmeal or sauté apples, can be used as a cooking medium, can be spread on chapattis or toast, directly nourishes *shukra dhatu* and increases *ojas*.

All of these habits can help decrease the *vata* that accumulates daily. We become our own master when we understand the qualities that throw *vata* off balance. Remember, *vata* has the qualities of being light, dry, cold, and mobile. If we keep these qualities in mind, we can step back and examine our lifestyle to make sure we are keeping any harmful activities to a minimum.

Pitta

Skin conditions and digestive complaints involving *pitta dosha* are the main imbalances which show up frequently in the clinic. Why? Because after a while, patients and parents run out of options. The steroids are no longer effective, the antibiotics seem to help tentatively, and patients are lost in terms of healthy food habits. Patients of all ages, from birth to middle age, seem to be plagued with *pitta*-related disease processes. The *pitta* stage of life begins around age 16. At this time, acne and a rebellious nature emerge. Though this is the *pitta* time of life, any disease can still take place based on causative factors and their duration. Below is a collection of case vignettes with vitiated *pitta dosha* as the main culprit.

Case Study 1: Kushtha (skin disorder)

A 34-yr-old male patient, 5'6" and weighing 180 lbs, walked into my office about three years ago. He sat down and showed me an abnormal patch of skin roughly the size of a quarter on his left thigh. As I uncovered his lifestyle and dietary factors, I came to find out that he had been consuming a typical south Indian specialty, yogurt and rice, every day for about two years. The dermatologist he had visited prior to seeing me had given him only one option—a topical steroid application. The patient knew that he needed to get to the root of his skin problem. This led him to consult with me and make the decision to begin down the path of *Ayurveda.* I probed a bit further and found other causative factors as well, such as exposure to the Arizona sun (which was new for him), stress through work, and intermittent travel. None of these compared in strength and duration to his daily consumption of yogurt.

His *doshas* had accumulated, particularly *pitta* and *kapha*, in *rakta dhatu*. We started with herbs and then we came to know that the load of *doshas* was too heavy for his body to handle. The rash started spreading to his right leg where a scar remained from an old surgery. Soon, even the other leg was affected. The excess *doshas* were lodged deep inside his tissues, and it was time to administer *panchakarma* detoxification treatments. We started with *vaman*, an emesis procedure, as we knew *kapha dosha* had a part to play in his illness. His *doshas* became aggravated and his skin got quite worse before getting better. In *Ayurveda*, this type of skin disease is called *Kushtha*. His skin became consumed by imbalanced *doshas*. Over a period of two years he received two *vamans*, two *virechans* (laxative treatments), intermittent local bloodletting, and the application of leeches. He continued his herbal regimen well after his skin healed. Today, he is completely cured and even his skin color has come back. What an amazing healing process he went through. I still remember when he got up from his chair after the first *vaman* and said, "I have so much energy I could go running." The *doshas* had been weighing him down.

From this example, it becomes apparent that even though the skin is affected externally, internal cleansing is what is really needed. The first step in internal cleansing is to locate the causative factors. Causative factors such as cheese, tomatoes, yogurt, and other *pitta* and *kapha* aggravating foods played a role in this patient's skin rash. While *pitta* and *kapha* are the two main culprits, *vata* is necessary for the migration of skin problems.

Case Study 2: Mukha Dushika (acne)

I also had the joy of working with a 23-year-old woman who presented with a recreational drug addiction. She ended up with a case of facial acne. This acne was painful and filled with toxins that created abscesses. She started treatment. Her first step was letting go of the drugs immediately. She was very committed, so letting go wasn't hard. She went through her first round of both *vaman* and *virechan*. The *vaman* treatment was quite an emotional treatment for her. She cried before the treatment even began. She was a strong, dedicated woman not afraid to do anything—my ideal patient. I grew to admire this patient. She put her trust in me and followed all of my suggestions.

Because this patient was adopted, we were unsure what accumulation of past *doshas* may have been passed to her in utero. It didn't matter because we were dedicated to moving these *doshas* out. She experienced some relief from the first treatment, but the breakouts just wouldn't stop. The acne covered her from face to neck, with a few lesions even spreading to her back. We continued with numerous bloodletting sessions and the application of leeches to move local toxins out. The following year we repeated another series of *vaman* and *virechan*. She saw some results, but she was still unhappy with the breakouts. Somehow, I was able to convince her to do a third round of treatments. We removed the remaining *doshas* and her breakouts stopped. It is apparent to her when she has gone off track. She has put in so much hard work, dedication, and trust. Because of this, she achieved optimal results along with a life changing experience.

This is an example of the accumulation we hold in our tissues. One of my teachers explained it to me very succinctly. She uses the analogy of internal cabinets. Have you ever tried to add more items to a cabinet that is already full? The cabinet becomes packed so tightly that when you try to close it, its contents bulge outward. Our bodies are similar. These cabinets exist within us. It could be *doshas*, *ama*, or a mix of the two. When we begin the *panchakarma* procedures, pockets of *doshas* are released. The load of *doshas* and the duration of causative factors, determine the need for repeated treatments.

Case Study 3: Rakta Dushti (vitiated blood)

In the Southwestern United States, Valley Fever is quite common. It is described as a fungal infection caused by *Coccidioides immitus*, an organism that lies in the desert soil, affecting the lungs. Common symptoms include a fever, rash, chest pain, and a cough.

I was fortunate to be able to treat a 52-year-old patient who came to see me after an initial visit to the Emergency Room. She told me that her symptoms began with severe chest pain which landed her in the ER where she was ultimately diagnosed with Valley Fever. An x-ray revealed a nodule occupying the left lobe of her lung. She was told her only treatment option was an IV antibiotic, which they administered immediately. When she arrived home, she consulted with me, and I took that opportunity to begin diagnosing her according to *Ayurvedic* principles. The term Valley Fever really didn't mean anything to me. I had to determine *doshic* imbalances and the *dhatus* affected.

She was plagued with an extremely uncomfortable full-body rash. According to *Ayurveda*, the origin of lung tissue is *rakta dhatu*. The strength of the lungs depends on the health of *rakta dhatu*, hence treatments should always be geared toward formation of good quality *rakta dhatu*. We can accomplish this by avoiding causative factors that have the ability to vitiate *rakta*. I immediately started treating her with internal herbs to reduce the heat that had collected in her blood tissue. Cilantro juice was chosen as a topical to help ease the itching, cool the skin, and settle the rash. She was feeling better in no time.

After having been struck by this illness, this patient has a propensity to collect *doshas* in the lungs. Therefore, *Ayurveda* has an important concept of *rasayana* therapy, or a series of rejuvenating treatments which strengthen weak *dhatus*. After cleansing *panchakarma* treatments, or the use of herbal remedies, there are many *rasayanas* that can be given. The restorative quality of the herbal remedies has a better chance of reaching their respective areas. One tried and true method to strengthen the lungs is to consume *Pippali* (Indian long pepper) medicated milk. She has been receiving *panchakarma* yearly and has had no recurrence of the western diagnosis of Valley Fever.

Case Study 4: Amla Pitta (heartburn)

In the case of heartburn, many patients limit treatment to the use of an antacid and the avoidance of some foods (such as chocolate, citrus, and spicy food). It goes much deeper than this. In *Ayurveda*, most digestive complaints have to be assessed in terms of *doshas*, *ama*, and *agni*. This should be accompanied by a tongue assessment and an abdominal exam. Without all of these tools, it would be hard to give patients relief.

I recall one 54-year-old female patient who came to me about seven years ago. Her symptoms included fatigue, weakness, digestive complaints, and sensitivity to stimuli. We began treatment and managed to soothe most of her symptoms. However, as other symptoms subsided she continually complained of a "sour gut." Until now she had received mild *virechan* treatments as well as a few series of *bastis* (enemas). It later dawned on me that *vaman* would be the treatment she would need. Upon completion of the *vaman* treatment, she experienced instant relief from her acidity, describing a 40% improvement. Sometimes *pitta* actually lies above the umbilicus, in the *kapha* area of the body. The patient had past exposure to heavy pesticides and toxic situations, which may have been at the root of this. It could also have been a lack in her digestive fire to process certain *doshas*, along with poor food choices. During the *vaman*, red lines of sputum were visible. My teacher taught me not to become frightened, as *pitta* can appear red when expelled. The patient now understands the value of this treatment and continues to receive *panchakarma* yearly.

Case Study 5: Rakta Dushti (vitiated blood)

A 60-year-old patient visited me with persistent redness of the face. She had a lifelong tendency to become red around the nose, especially with exposure to the sun. This time it was different. She felt that this time the redness was related to a hair dye she had used as the symptoms seemed to appear after its application. She participated in a three-day internal preparation with medicated bitter ghee, followed by bloodletting. She was also given internal herbs to help decrease the *pitta* in her body. The redness went away within a few weeks, and since then she has been very careful to stay clear of the causative factors that we discovered such as tomatoes, potato chips, and milk especially when combined with salt (as in the kitchari she had been preparing regularly mixed with milk), as well as exposure to direct sunlight, toxic hair dye, and an open flame (as used for cooking). She was unaware of these causative factors until we were able to identify, treat, and avoid them for a total remission of 70-80% of the patient's symptoms.

Kapha

How would your life change if your kids rarely got sick? Sick days would become nonexistent, saving you from missing work or having to make last-minute child-care arrangements. It is likely that you or your children suffer chronically from one or more of the following symptoms: an opaque green, white, or yellow nasal discharge, achy ears, weakness, stomach discomfort, sinus pressure, or a low-grade fever. What is our go-to with such conditions? Typically, we first reach for antibiotics. I once rotated with a primary care doctor and we were bombarded with the symptoms above. It was to the patient's savior that if the illness were grouped into a viral category then an antibiotic would not be prescribed. We instructed those patients with a viral illness to drink fluids and rest. Common sense, one would think. This gave the patient's body a chance to heal on its own. The more we treat these conditions with antibiotics, the more we suppress the body from clearing disease on its own, causing the tissues to begin to weaken. Most of us have very little knowledge about a more natural approach to health, one that doesn't include popping a pill. Thankfully, the movement towards treating these problems naturally is gaining great momentum. This is where *Ayurveda* enters the picture as a guide on such matters.

I bet you are trying to understand what sets us up for these issues. Here are a few causative factors that may not be immediately obvious: bananas, yogurt with fruit, cold milk with cereal, avocados, and cheese.

What do these foods have in common? They are cold, sticky, and predominantly made of earth and water elements (which aggravates *kapha dosha*). The consistent intake of cold and sticky food choices hampers our digestive fire, which in turn creates ama. Until I began to study *Ayurveda*, I didn't understand the effect these foods have on our being either. The quality that each food exhibits is what is important.

Kapha has other qualities as well, including being stable, oily, heavy, cloudy, gross, dull, slow, and smooth. *Kapha's* physiologic function is to provide structure, strength, and immunity to our being.

From birth until age 16, we enter into the *kapha* stage of life. Recall any newborn baby. The baby isn't aware of these qualities, but those around the baby will surely pick up on them: overflowing love, joy, and supple skin, to name a few.

What course of action should we take to mitigate these recurrent infections? We should start by avoiding the causative factors that increase *kapha* in the body. *Kapha* predominantly resides in the upper third of the body, which is where most respiratory conditions occur. Therefore, the foods mentioned above should be avoided. Of course, milk can be ingested, but it should be boiled for better digestion. It is common in our culture to give kids cold milk with cereal. The cold quality of the milk, as well as the fact that most cereals have salt (which doesn't combine well with milk) adds to our *doshic* load. Not to worry—I grew up having sugary cereals and milk as well, until I was taught otherwise. I have built relationships with my favorite breakfast cereals, whether Cinnamon Toast Crunch, Lucky Charms, or Fruity Pebbles. If left to my own devices, I could have eaten cereal for breakfast, lunch, and dinner.

Keeping our channels healthy in order to build stronger tissues is the key. Healthy tissue building starts from a young age. Again, I recall my teacher's words, as she once explained that Veda would love the healthy food I offer to her as she would not know what she was missing in regards to cheese, tomatoes, and other *kaphic*, non-*sattvic* foods. This is the time to build healthy tissues and keep the digestive fire kindled.

Fevers are another common issue plaguing both kids and adults. How does *Ayurveda* describe febrile conditions? It begins with *ama*, which is any material that has not been properly digested. *Ama* begins to travel into the first tissue of the body (known as *rasa dhatu*). As a result, a fever develops. The treatment for fevers are quite simple. The main goal is to simply fast until the fever has passed. This fasting is termed as *langhana*. They were onto something with that old myth of starving a fever. Thin, liquid rice water is allowed if one feels extremely weak or hungry. In modern medicine, we treat a fever as a symptom, but in *Ayurveda*, fever is a disease in and of itself. It is actually one of the first diseases we cover in understanding the disease process. The principles set forth by *Charaka* regarding *ama*, fasting, and *doshas* create the perfect lens through which to view how other disease processes ensue.

I have numerous patients who come to me complaining of recurrent sinus infections. Recall back to the sticky, white, drying, cold, and congestive foods we discussed earlier. One of the first things I ask about is their consumption of bananas. Quite often, a patient will tell me they consume one or more bananas every day. I was surprised at first, but have now become accustomed to it. I ask them to avoid bananas for two weeks and roughly 60% of their symptoms improve. Bananas have the capacity to clog up the channels, aggravating both *vata* and *kapha*. I ask everyone to avoid them in general. *Vata* and *kapha* live in the sinus cavities. When too much *kapha* begins to accumulate in these spaces, symptoms begin showing up.

Once again, the first line of treatment is to avoid the causative factors, but the healing doesn't stop there. What about the remaining *doshas* that accumulated prior to stopping the causative factors? We have taken care to see that the *doshas* don't accumulate any further, but we must eradicate what has collected. This happens with the help of herbs, other treatments, or *panchakarma* (if the load is quite heavy). One of the simplest ways to treat blocked sinus cavities is with the use of salt, oil, and steam. One should mix warm oil and salt together and apply over the sinuses. Then expose the sinuses to steam for 5-10 minutes. The salt breaks the *kapha* apart, the oil pacifies the *vata*, and the steam helps open up the channels. I love that this medicine always makes sense intuitively. It's the beauty of having the entire universe as our pharmacy. Until we begin to become curious about the elements in nature and study their impact on the *doshas*, we will not understand our inner nature.

CHAPTER FIVE

Brave *Moves*

I grew up immersed in various art forms. From the young age of eight, I found myself participating in Indian folk and classical dancing, Indian classical singing, and even playing an Indian instrument called the harmonium. A solo debut performance in front of a large audience at age 18 illustrates a transformation that occurred. My nerves were silently screaming with unchanneled *vata*. I was able to harness these nerves as I began dancing joyfully and with heartfelt expression. Today, as I gaze into my daughter's eyes I am reminded of that expression of joy, which she communicates through her exuberant movements. This was a pivotal point in my life as this courageous experience set the stage for my future endeavors.

I went on to complete my bachelor's degree at a liberal arts school, American University, in Washington, DC. It was so ironic. While everyone else dove into business, literature, or graphic design, only 12 other students and I chose a path in chemistry. What are the chances? It's no coincidence that I chose such a path. I always had to be unique. I began my studies and knew that with my parents and grandparents being doctors, I too would focus my work in the health field. I was exposed to and surrounded by a broad spectrum of disciplines in medicine such as psychiatry, emergency medicine, obstetrics, and surgery, beginning at a young age.

I chose chemistry as my pre-medical major. In order to graduate, a certain number of liberal arts classes were mandatory. My attention was drawn to a series of philosophy classes, even prompting me to consider minoring in it. Hobbes, Locke, Thoreau, Machiavelli, and Socrates are just a few of the great philosophers I studied. The *Oxford Dictionary* defines philosophy *as the study of the fundamental nature of knowledge, reality, and existence.* The word philosophy comes from the Ancient Greek *philosophia,* which literally means *love of wisdom.*

It is clear to me now that my curiosity was rooted in discovering not only how the world came to be, but how this perfect mixture of organic and inorganic matter combined to create life. I had come full circle. A mix of science, philosophy, and medicine was the fullest expression of these art forms. This is the essence of *Ayurveda: the science and art of living life.*

This led me to a career in medicine, but my focus was on medicine from a naturopathic perspective. I always thought I would go onto allopathic school, but I listened to my heart. It was my guiding force. I had always loved pondering the inner workings of both nature and the human body. I recall a common question I had as a child—why don't human beings need an external source of electricity in order to function? Human anatomy and physiology were always so interesting.

I attended Bastyr University, another naturopathic school, for a summer, and started my studies in Chinese medicine and Thai massage. This confirmed my career path, as I settled on a school in Arizona to begin my journey.

After four grueling years, I had learned all there was to know about acupuncture, western herbs, homeopathy, nutrition (from a macronutrient point of view), physical medicine, environmental medicine, and much more. Can you believe my mind and body were still left unfulfilled? I was empty and waiting to fill up again. I graduated, still unsure of myself. I seemed to be missing a unifying system to help me integrate the myriad of treatments I had begun to practice. I needed to continue learning and get much closer to my roots.

My parents and grandparents were born and raised in East Africa, while I was born in the United Kingdom. As I've mentioned before, I was surrounded by a family of physicians. Although I had been exposed to modern, western medicine, my heart still yearned to explore more about life and disease through a naturalistic lens. I feel very fortunate to have come upon *Ayurvedic* medicine, and I am grateful to all my mentors on this path.

My journey started with Dr. Paul Dugliss, who introduced me to Dr. Suhas. From there, I met Dr. Yash Mannur, Dr. Rasik, Dr. Gadgil, and Dr. Vedhas. I was searching for authentic teachings and the ability to read and translate directly from the scriptures written by *Charaka*, *Sushruta*, and *Vagbhata*. I immersed myself in the teachings of these three scholars. One mentor led me to the next. It's as if I needed to dig deeper and reconnect with my roots. As I came to know more about *Ayurvedic* medicine, I learned that *Ayurveda* and yoga were sister sciences, and I needed to pursue them both. I completed a yoga teacher certification with another one of my amazing gurus, Jonny Kest. His training taught me all the ins and outs of yoga, learning to reach my edge, and learning to be present with an underlying foundation of *Vipassana* meditation.

Dr. Paul Dugliss was an internal medicine doctor back in Michigan, my hometown, with whom my grandfather once consulted. I am indebted to him and feel that meeting him was my first step on this path. He was part of the *Maharishi* movement at one point, and I partook in his first official class. He taught me the basics of *Ayurveda*, which was just what I needed to allow this science to integrate into my cells and fill the emptiness. He led us to Hawaii, where I learned various hands-on therapies, including *abhyanga* (oil massage).

The program in Hawaii was spearheaded by Dr. Suhas. He added a layer of *Vedic* astrology to my training, as well as further training back on the mainland with a program he was later affiliated with called Kerala Ayurveda Academy, based in Fremont. My mom and I traveled to Fremont, CA monthly to complete that program. I kept falling deeper and deeper in love with this science. It was at this point when I met Dr. Yash Mannur. I implored her to take me under her wing and teach me even more. I learned from wonderful scholars and became dedicated to this knowledge with the understanding that my true healing would begin here. I learned from Dr. Rasik, Dr. Vedas, and Dr. Gadgil, all of whom traveled from India regularly to teach us.

In order to join the program Dr. Yash was running, I had to catch up with her first year students. With the help of a dear classmate, I passed the first year tests with flying colors, confidently able to demonstrate what I learned. This allowed me to join Dr. Yash and her students in India for an internship. I had a wonderful time in India, learning from the heart of it all. We visited factories where herbs were being produced. I saw, felt, and tasted raw herbs before they were formulated, watched authentic *panchakarma* treatments, and immersed myself completely. I felt fortunate after having returned from India. I traveled back and forth between home and Fremont, ultimately completing my second year at the Shubham Ayurveda Clinic.

The knowledge I acquired during this period was everything I needed to formulate a healthy path forward for my studies and my life. Even today, I continue to listen to all of the live lectures, which honor and carry on the tradition of *Ayurveda*. I continue to peel back layer after layer of this ancient wisdom daily. *Ayurveda* is oceans deep. My love for this science will go on for a lifetime and far beyond. This is my true calling. Being able to bring these teachings to the United States and practice with my naturopathic foundation has given me the ability to be a physician and an *Ayurvedic* practitioner.

CHAPTER SIX

A Peek Within

At the culmination of my fourth year of naturopathic medical school, I was getting ready to take my final clinical board exams. I was studying with a few friends at Barnes and Noble, when I took a break and visited the restroom. As I finished washing my hands, I caught a glimpse of myself in the mirror which caused me to do a double take—I was missing a chunk of hair. I arrived home quickly that night and ran a comb through my hair to determine if there were any other sparse areas, and indeed there were. The stress I'd been experiencing had finally caught up with me. We have all been there: endless studying with caffeine as our primary motivation, managing the complexities of romance, neglecting exercise due to packed schedules, and improper food choices. Ultimately, I made it through my exams and was happily married a year later.

My husband, my family, and I started eating out quite a bit. My husband and I were notorious for ordering Papa John's once a week, savoring the sinful goodness of a pizza topped with jalapeños, onions, green peppers, and pineapples. Their side of garlic butter sauce was a must. I simply wasn't paying attention. Post-marriage, I began to pack on the weight, to the tune of roughly 10 lbs a year. At the time, it wasn't obvious how far off track I was. Looking back, it seemed to have happened overnight. Before I knew it, I was 180 lbs. My periods were growing further and further apart. I knew something had to change. My journey inward began, and I enthusiastically enrolled in an authentic *Ayurvedic* education program in Fremont, California. My own healing process coincided with my growing knowledge of *Ayurveda*. Dr. Yash and Dr. Rasik met me for a consultation. Somehow, my periods had stopped for about four months. The doctors handed me a packet of herbs and told me with such confidence that on day eight of taking these herbs, my periods would return. I recall inquiring about the herbs and was informed that Dr. Rasik had prescribed *Kumari*, commonly known as Aloe vera. His instructions were to take the herbs twice a day with a glass of warm milk, once before lunch, and once again before dinner. Lo and behold, eight days later he was proven completely right. I was amazed by the results and had become convinced.

Dr. Yash had been seeing me prior to me taking these herbs. She is my mentor, my guru, and my lifelong friend. There was an occasion when we met face-to-face, and from mere observation, which is key in *Ayurveda*, she remarked that my face resembled a hormonal face. She got it. The science of *Ayurveda* was right on. I started a series of *bastis*, or enemas so my periods would start regulating. I never questioned her instructions. I gave up bread, tomatoes, and cheese. Second and third to pizza were my love for toast with chai and a delicious plate of nachos smothered in cheese and beans. This was a favorite lunch option for my sisters and I, a signature dish; we would go for seconds and thirds as we devoured them straight from the tray. Not just any cheese—sharp cheddar cheese. Not just any chai with bread—toasted wheat bread smothered with ghee and dipped just-so into the chai tea, retaining a perfect ratio of softness to crunch. Actually, the combination of tea and toast is very common in England, where I was born. I gave up what we call *hetus,* or causative factors. My main disease process involved *meda* (fat tissue) and *vata.* Excess *meda dhatu* was blocking my *vata* from flowing. The treatment involved avoiding *meda* aggravating foods, melting the *meda,* thus allowing *vata* to flow again.

My first step was to eliminate the causative factors. My load began to lighten immediately. I started the treatments both to continue my own personal healing, as well as prepare my body for pregnancy. By this time in my training, I had witnessed five or six *vaman* treatments, which is medical emesis. Because we took the unusual step of planning our pregnancy, my husband and I knew this same treatment was in store for both of us. We knew that until we had cleansed internally, a baby was not what the doctor had ordered. Yagnesh had a history of skin problems from his use of tobacco. We knew the best thing we could do to ensure a healthy future for our family would be to start clean. We didn't hesitate and soon braved the *vaman* procedure. The *vaman* procedure consisted of consuming increasing amounts of ghee over the course of seven days, followed by a day of fasting, and finally, emesis. Each evening we received *abhyanga* massage and steam, which made the experience all the more relaxing. I just knew that I had to take this one day at a time. I kept my goals and hopes for the future close to my heart and mind in order to remind myself to keep going. I had to cleanse the past in order to bring a new being into our lives.

I will admit, during the *vaman*, some fear about the idea of throwing up began to surface. I always hated it as a kid. Questions in my head arose: Could I do it? Did I have the strength? I clung to the knowledge that in order to administer this treatment to patients in the future I must first experience it myself. I had to be strong. After seven days of medicated ghee intake, I knew that it had done its job of creating a barrier and protecting the good tissues from any toxic junk that had accumulated. The ghee acted as a lubricant allowing the *doshas* to slide out. The night before the actual *vaman* treatment, after the seven-day intake of ghee, but before the actual emesis began, we visited an Indian restaurant. We were allowed to eat a combination of yogurt and rice, a typical snack called *dahi vada*, prescribed to create an increase in *kapha dosha*. That night, my sleep was uneasy. I had seen the treatment applied before, but now I had to gain the courage to do it myself. My teacher came into town to supervise the day of *vaman*. A wonderful helper, Disha, stayed with us for the week in order to help us in preparing food, as well as to monitor our daily progress. We seemed to get into quite a rhythm. I counted on them throughout the process.

The actual *vaman* day approached. The *Dhanvantari* prayer was performed at 6 am. The treatment had begun. It was time to drink the decoction. No one could do it for me. My husband and I sat next to one another, buckets on hand. I started drinking a pre-made licorice decoction. The *doshas* started to purge out on their own. Beginning with the upper stomach, emerging into the mouth, and out into the bucket. I couldn't believe what I was seeing. White, thick strands, frothy in nature and containing no food or smell, just *doshas* combined with the decoction, bout after bout. I was sweating. My guts were hurting from the inside out. The medicine went deep inside to scoop out the *doshas*. I had to keep going. My vision was in sight. I was doing this for our future. My husband was doing so well next to me. Actually, an hour passed by and he was done. I couldn't believe it. I started to lose my drive. I took a short break to sit back, breathe deeply, and give myself a small pep-talk. My mom was behind me, giving me the support I needed. My uncle was Yagnesh's support. Yagnesh had left the room. It was up to me to finish. Somehow, I gained the strength to pull through. As I called upon the universe to help me, an image of my grandmother came to me. I started gulping one glass of decoction after another, and before I knew it, I was done.

I sat back and took a deep breath as I gazed into the tub of *doshas* I had collected. I put a glove on, reached inside the tub, and rubbed my index finger and thumb together, examining the quality of what had been purged out. There was a thick, white layer of *kapha* that appeared on top of a brown layer of licorice decoction. My childhood flashed before my eyes. I was instantly reminded of my love for *kaphic* foods including cake. Not just any cake, Entenmann's pound cake dipped in milk. I also had flashes of Coke floats (Coca-Cola with a scoop of vanilla ice cream) and trifle (a layered dessert featuring jello, custard, cake, whipped cream, and fruit). I was astounded that evidence of poor dietary choices so far in my past was still able to surface and be purged.

The human body is amazing. Its capacity for collecting toxins seems limitless. But one can only continue accumulating toxins for so long until symptoms start to surface. This is the information I gathered. After the *vaman* was complete, I spent four days on a rice water drink to bring my digestive fire back. My husband and I rested and recovered. When I finally weighed myself, I discovered I had lost a total of 12 lbs, even though weight isn't a parameter, and never would be, as my teachers have taught me. My entire physiology started to change. I had actually lost about 7 lbs pounds after the seven days of ghee intake. *Doshas* had already begun to leave their cozy homes. My periods were taking shape. Thus began my journey of cleansing.

Following *vaman*, I continued with *virechan*, a laxative treatment. *Virechan* uses the same preparation of ghee, but this time *pitta dosha* is purged out. These treatments were followed with *basti* (a series of enemas) and lastly, a vaginal ghee preparation. I actually went to Fremont to get the last few treatments. Because of the amount of *kapha* that still resided within me, my teacher used a scraping method in administering the *bastis*. Even though my cleansing was apparently complete, I was unable to conceive for a few months. I was still nauseated daily, a sign that there were still unexpected *doshas* remaining. I continued to prepare for another *vaman* treatment. I quickly learned that no one can tell what is in store for another being. My body wanted to throw out more *doshas*. I didn't question it. Again, I just did what was necessary. I was committed to this process. I set up for another *vaman*, this time alongside my sister. The treatment went well, and I was now cleansed. I even continued one more series of *basti* treatments after this. Just when I least expected it, I became pregnant. The *panchakarma* treatments my husband and I underwent had paved the way for this new being to come into our lives.

I continued with *Ayurvedic* medicines throughout my pregnancy. I was under a midwife's care. She had a lot of advice about nutrition and various other recommendations, but I tried to blend my knowledge with that of the midwife's. I went to birthing classes with my husband. He was supportive of everything. I remember how stressful it had been, knowing that there was this new life growing inside me, and that I had to always do my best, as my every action had an effect on the baby, but I managed nonetheless. We did everything we could to prepare for this bundle of joy, including two different birthing classes. One was called *Birthing from Within*, a more spiritually based practice, while the other, *The Bradley Method*, was based in traditional practices. I wanted as much knowledge as possible. I even followed the prescribed methods of *Ayurveda* during my pregnancy. During the last month, I did some oil *bastis*, meant to assist with a smooth delivery as well as ease the *vata* that accumulates during pregnancy.

Finally, the moment I had been waiting for arrived. Veda was born exactly three hours after her due date. Everything went as planned. Little did I know, it would be a five-day affair. Our hard work, the pre-natal detoxing, the tears, the confusion, and the waiting, had all paid off with the arrival of Veda. I had been preparing my whole life for this moment. It was in my hands. I remember having a significant breakthrough the day before Veda arrived. Fear and failure began to invade the tiny spaces in my mind as the universe and its divine timing gave me all of my answers. I felt deeply supported by both my mother and Mother Nature. I felt so grateful for this experience in my life. It has shaped the person I am today. It showed me that anything is possible. I do have the strength. The actual *panchakarma* was just a precursor. This was the *peek within* that I needed to understand that if I can withstand *vaman*, then I can deliver naturally. If I can deliver naturally, then I can write a book, and so on.

CHAPTER SEVEN

Principles Of The Universe

The theory of *karana* (cause) and *karya* (effect) is one of the most important concepts in *Ayurveda*. *Charaka* has described cause and effect in reference to health and disease conditions. Understanding the concept of cause and effect helps achieve the ultimate goal of *Ayurveda*, which is the maintenance of health and the curing of disease in affected individuals. Everything in the universe follows this theory. Some(thing) precedes the effect. Therefore, we must always examine what that is, especially if it has a negative effect.

Another universal principle found in *Ayurveda* is that everything in the universe can be broken down into the five elements: space, air, fire, water, and earth.

Finally, the ancient texts of *Ayurveda* list the twenty *gunas* or ten pairs of opposites. *Guna* is a Sanskrit word which translates into attribute or quality. Theoretically, everything in the universe can be described in terms of these qualities. *Gunas* can be associated with each element, *dosha*, symptom, food, yoga pose, and mood. They are extremely important to identify as they are fundamental in developing a treatment plan. We must identify imbalanced *gunas* and treat

accordingly. For example, it is common to think that the opposite of dry is wet but, in fact, it is oily. The 10 pairs of *gunas*
are listed below:

Heavy - Light
Cold - Hot
Static - Mobile
Soft - Hard
Oily - Dry
Transparent - Opaque
Dull - Sharp
Smooth - Rough
Gross - Subtle
Dense - Liquid

What is Medicine?

What exactly qualifies as medicine? Growing up, the
pink bubble-gum flavored amoxicillin was always present
in the fridge. But, as I have grown wiser, I now understand
that medicine exists all around us. Our entire universe is our
medicinal pharmacy—plants, food, dancing, music, babies,
and making love to name a few. To me, medicine is anything
that allows our body to heal and has the ability to counteract
negative forces in the body, bringing us into balance.

Pharmaceuticals have their role. We have come to understand that they too have their own *gunas*, which are mostly
bitter, aggravating *vata dosha*. Birth control pills or topical
creams tend to aggravate the blood tissue and push the *doshas* further into our tissues. Patients have told me that they
see the benefit of topicals and admit that it is an easier option. We are still stuck in that mindset. We don't have the

patience to understand that if the disease is of x duration, it will then take x amount of years to cure. We are trying to get rid of complex disease processes that have come to a head over time. The western medical definition of health lies in the mere absence of disease. *Ayurveda's* definition of health travels much further, as written below in Sanskrit:

Swasthasya Swaasthya Rakshanam

Aaturasya Vikara Prashamanam Cha

(Charaka Samhita-Sutra Sthana 30/26)

This translation states that the aim of *Ayurveda* is to protect the health of the healthy and help rid the suffering of the sufferer. *Ayurveda* emphasizes *prevention*. It not only helps us regain our health by eliminating the root cause of illness, but also has numerous dietary and lifestyle recommendations to be followed daily in order to prevent disease.

Our life expectancy and health depend on three pillars: *ahara* (diet), *nidra* (sleep), and *brahmacharya* (balanced sexual drive). *Charaka Samhita*, the ancient authoritative text of *Ayurveda*, has given due importance to them.

The Disease Process

Doshas accumulate due to the causative factors that are present. *Vata* is responsible for almost 80% of all disease because it's the only *dosha* that can actually move the other stable *doshas, pitta* and *kapha.* Elsewhere there is a *dhatu* (tissue), *srotas* (channel), or *avayava* (organ) that is weak. This could be due to the recurrent use of a certain area of the body or recurrent infections. The *doshas* that have accumulated start to find shelter in one of these weakened areas and start to wreak havoc there. When this interaction takes place, disease is formed. Until then, it's just a set of symptoms. Once *doshas* have been pacified with the help of herbs or removed from the body via *panchakarma* detoxification treatments, the *dhatu* (or tissue) itself must be strengthened so that the *doshas* don't take shelter there again. There are certain correlations of which to be aware. *Vata* takes shelter more easily in the bones, *pitta* more easily in the blood tissue, and *kapha* more easily in the joints. The only way to reverse this process is to identify the causative factors and avoid them. Then, we must separate the *doshas* from the *dhatus* which breaks the chain of disease. We continue by strengthening the weak space where the *doshas* initially found a home.

Panchakarma Basics

I feel fortunate to not only provide *bastis* to my patients, but to be able to administer *vaman*, *virechan*, and various forms of blood-letting according to the ancient tradition. I have personally undergone these treatments. I have also taken many patients through these treatments and have seen miracles occur. One way to think of *panchakarma* is that it is equivalent to microsurgery of the body that doesn't require an incision. How can surgery be performed without the use of a sharp instrument? How can a substance with such opposite nature, such as ghee, sharply separate the good tissues from the toxic *doshas?* The medicated ghee is used due to its bitter nature. The bitter quality has the ability to travel into the smallest channels and perform this separation process.

Panchakarma translates into five actions, which consist of *vaman, virechan, basti, nasya,* and *raktamokshan.* The purpose of *panchakarma* is to remove chunks of *doshas* which at times can be much faster than the use of herbs. These *karmas* purge *vata, pitta, kapha,* and vitiated *rakta* out of the body through the closest track available. *Vaman* is the emesis procedure and involves assisted vomiting. *Virechan* is a laxative treatment, and *basti* involves the use of nourishing and cleansing enemas. People often ask me how *bastis* differ from colonics. *Bastis* effects are more widespread helping remove the vitiated *doshas* from all over the body while preserving the good tissues. Colonics, on the other hand, work locally to remove the toxic material from the colon only, but fail to replenish and nourish the system in order to take care of the excess movement created to pull out the toxins. I have seen amazing results from *panchakarma* procedures for all types of conditions, including skin, heartburn, and infertility.

I feel grateful to have been taught the procedures listed above in a very authentic manner. These treatments are not offered very often here in the United States. Rather, in India, there are *Ayurvedic* hospitals where these treatments are performed. I had a chance to do an internship in Pune, India as part of my training, and I was able to watch and assist patients undergoing a variety of *panchakarma* procedures. I was amazed at my time there. There are a number of people with access to such treatments. It is my fortune that I can administer these safely here in the United States.

Healing and detoxification is accessible to us all. The rewards are great. It is our misunderstanding that we think we have to constantly rid the body of defilements. The term *detoxification* has become so common, but we fail to consider the need to nourish our system. *Ayurveda* has thought of everything. One of my core naturopathic principles is to first do no harm. The pre-*panchakarma* procedure sums this up very well. All of the five *karmas* begin with an internal and external oleation process. This involves being careful to protect good tissues so that the *doshas* can flow out easier. The aforementioned medicated ghee functions to separate the non-toxic from the toxic. Everyone must continue some form of *panchakarma* once a year. It is equivalent to giving your car an oil change. We collect *doshas* just from living life, and cleansing is a necessary part of the flow of life. When we observe Mother Nature, we notice it follows a similar trend. Natural disasters, such as tsunamis, forest fires, and earthquakes are evidence of *doshic* imbalance. My interpretation is that this is the universe's way of purging the *doshic* load that has become too high in order to maintain homeostasis.

Breaking Down My Health Journey

Looking back, I can see that my journey was a step-by-step process. There were peaks and valleys. Locating the causative factors is the first step when evaluating a patient. If we fail to locate and eliminate them, our system will continue to accumulate *doshas* while simultaneously trying to move *doshas* out or pacify them. In my situation, stress and *kaphic* food choices were my causative factors. What does stress mean? It is such a general term. Stress can affect the *doshas* in different ways. Generally, it affects *vata* the most and it manifests as constant worry, fear, or overthinking. In terms of *Ayurveda*, the excess vata tends to dry out our mental sphere. There is a word for it—*chinta*. Can you imagine chronically using your mind more than it wants to be used? This is one of the most common cultivators of disease. We need to let go of this worry, fear, and constant thinking. For me, stress manifested first as hair loss.

Vata is responsible for the monthly cycles through its downward movement. Because *doshas* were blocking the path, my periods were very painful when they started coming back. Pain is always associated with *vata dosha*. I eliminated my major food aggravators such as cheese, milk combined with salt, tomatoes, and bread, mostly because they were blocking the flow in my body. I started the *vaman panchakarma* procedure when my body and mind were mentally prepared. I had already seen a difference with the herbs and a few *bastis* here and there, but more had to be done due to the duration of both the causative factors and the symptoms themselves. This is when *panchakarma* is precisely indicated—when there has been excess nourishment that the body has received. I was packing on excess pounds; my face had ballooned up, a typical sign of *vata* being out of balance. I would have been diagnosed with Polycystic Ovarian Syndrome from a western perspective. I knew I could handle my disease process using *Ayurvedic* methods. It was time to make a change. After the detox programs, I decided to also eliminate meat and alcohol. These substances are *ojas* and *sattvic* depleting substances, which interfere in our ability to tune in more deeply to our being.

A *sattvic* individual is one who is divine, pure, spiritual, and keeps practices to remain in that state. From the moment of conception, a baby receives all its nourishment from its mother. Therefore, it is important for the mother to remain as *sattvic* as possible so that the baby receives purity at each step of its development. In addition, the mother's daily mental attitude plays a vital role. I participated in a ten-day noble silent *Vipassana* meditation retreat during the fifth month of pregnancy to help facilitate a peaceful, loving, and compassionate mind. It took me three years to regain my health. I feel fortunate to have had the guidance to plan and prepare for conception.

Pregnancy

According to *Ayurveda*, we should strive to have the healthiest child possible. Per *Ayurveda*, childbearing should be complete by age 25. The mental imprint of the child from conception to birth should be of *sattva guna*—purity, pleasure, and happiness. *Shukra*, the reproductive tissue, is associated with creativity, contentment, and pleasure. Intercourse has become emotionless as couples are bombarded by the stress of conceiving resulting in infertility which plagues our culture now. In *Ayurveda*, there are medicines that help with fertility, but only after cleansing is performed through *panchakarma*. We should be doing our best to create quality children, generation after generation. My belief is that future generations deserve the best. We must decrease our load in order to give to the future. That means detoxing the body, moving into those sticky layers, and clearing the path for both man and woman. Both partner's *doshic* load is carried into the next generation. Repeated miscarriages are the body's way of telling us that the body is under stress. Why not give it a break by cleansing, de-stressing, and living in accordance with nature's rhythms.

Sattva, Rajas, and Tamas

Rajas is defined by the *guna* of activity or fire. *Tamasic* energy is dark, heavy, and clouded. Our main goal is to venture toward a *sattvic* lifestyle by keeping with the times of waking and sleeping, consuming *sattvic* foods, and partaking in *sattvic* activities.

Alcohol is one of the substances that takes us away from leading a *sattvic* life. It is known that alcohol has qualities opposite to the qualities of *ojas*. It is a poison that is *rajasic* in nature with an ability to permeate the tissues quickly, travel straight to the heart, and harbor disease. It slowly brings us away from developing *sattvic* qualities, which we need to strengthen our mental disposition in order to ward off mental illness such as depression and anxiety. Mental *doshas* of *vata*, *pitta*, and *kapha* do exist. They start bothering us when the foundation of the mind is weak. Therefore, it is important to keep anything that brings us away from this *sattvic* nature at a minimum.

Meat is another contributing factor that allows for decreased *sattva guna*. I am often asked whether *Ayurveda* insists on the necessity of a vegetarian diet. *Ayurveda* stresses the importance of this in order to keep *sattva guna* working at its best. The consumption of meat brings us away from developing *sattvic* qualities, because we don't know the mental state of the animal at the time of its death. That mental state adds to our already shattered state. Additionally, meat is very heavy for digestion. Red meat is especially sticky, having the tendency to hamper digestion. We must always dig deeper to better understand the *gunas* of each substance. As we gain a better knowledge of the *gunas*, we can begin to answer our own questions.

CHAPTER EIGHT

A Day At An Ayurvedic Clinic

As a doctor, an *Ayurvedic* practitioner, and a patient myself, I regularly stand at the clinic gates and recall its birth, as every property whether inhabited or not has its own unique story. The energy pouring out onto 1st avenue through the gated fence has a way of inviting the passerby. The gate spans the property as a way to protect the courtyard. A gracious eucalyptus tree stands tall in the center of the courtyard. One cannot smell the scent of the eucalyptus immediately, but once the leaves are rubbed or even used in water to create steam for lung treatments, the properties of this medicinal oil are unleashed.

As the rustic gates are pushed open, the original red bricks pave the walkway, and a rose garden blooms in season. Ceramic pots overflow with yellow lantanas and a couple of cozy, refurbished rocking chairs invite guests. A path leads down the eastern part of the property and is lined with statues of *Ganesha, Saraswati*, and *Buddha*. All of these statues have found a home, not for any religious purpose, but because of the qualities they possess. *Ganesha* is known for removing obstacles, *Saraswati* is known for her ability to impart knowledge, music, arts, wisdom, and learning, and *Buddha* is known for exuding loving compassion. This courtyard is one of the reasons we were drawn to acquire this property, as courtyards have their significance dating back to 6400 BC and are very common in Indian architecture. Courtyards offer a sense of comfort where community can gather, as well as a way to turn inward and connect with nature.

A small, slightly recessed 2600-square-foot home built in the 1920's stands in the middle of the property. A long and colorful history predates our ownership of the property. Horses used to be tied up to a long, half-rotten, wooden post studded with large silver rings. The posts were removed a few years back and replaced by the rose garden. A few patients have told me that they had a member of their family tie their horses to this property while visiting the old optometry building which is now a juice bar. We have kept the building in its exact form with very few changes.

Sacred chants and a beautiful wind chime accompany nature's sounds. As one walks down the path on the east side of the building there is the opportunity to ring a bell that hangs just as one would prior to entering a temple. Why east? Because the sun rises in the east, allowing the most beneficial energy to activate the property. This entrance cultivates feelings of safety, which is foundational for anyone on a healing path. The original solid, knotted oak floor remains, bringing alive *kaphic* energy as one enters the clinic.

We are located on 1st avenue in the heart of Old Town Scottsdale, Arizona surrounded by recently built lofts, Kaleidoscope Juice, Grimaldi's Pizza, Bicycle Haus, and the Sugar Bowl. 1st avenue is changing—out with the old and in with the new. People love to come and sit, soaking up the energy in the shade of the eucalyptus tree on warm days, and basking in the sunlight on cold Arizona winter days. Buildings left and right are being renovated, creating a modern landscape that mixes with the ancient energy that seeps from the cracks of our 100-year-old building.

Some may wonder what it is that takes place in this small recessed home. Some commonly asked questions are: *Do you sell statues? Can I take photographs? Are you a gallery? Can I just hang out?* I typically see patients by appointment, but on the off chance that the clinic is open, people wander in, drawn to the energy. We are all seeking connection, a place that makes us feel safe and is willing to hold our hand on this journey.

Patients, therapists, and those merely strolling by all wait at the gate, observing what it is that's tugging at their heart, speaking to their emotional body, and settling their mind. Immediately the vibration of the relics, sounds, and nature create a positive space to nullify the negativity present in a person's being. We often take nature for granted. We forget that it is constantly supporting us as long as we are aware.

Into the Therapeutic Process

We take in the world through our five senses: touch, taste, smell, sound, and vision. As one enters the clinic, all five are enlivened in one form or another.

TOUCH

As one makes their way into the therapy room, labeled the *freedom to receive* room, the client is invited to disrobe and lie down on the table. Bamboo lines the ceiling as a focal point for the client's eyes to rest. Our signature two-person *abhyanga* oil massage precedes all detoxification procedures. The chanting of three *"oms"* allows the patient and therapists to connect. This is followed by an invocation of *Lord Dhanvantari*. The magic of *Ayurveda* begins to fill the room. We all want to feel loved, and we crave connection daily. The dance begins as warm oil is drizzled onto every part of the body. This process keeps us coming back for more.

What is it about touch? Skin is the sense organ related to air, which pacifies *vata*. Can you imagine four synchronized hands providing gentle strokes to each body part? Care at the deepest level is attained through stimulating the hair follicles, massaging the ear lobes, and applying pressure on *marma* points which exist throughout the body. The patient melts into the table as the warmth and density of the oil is grounding. The patient is able to surrender, allowing stillness and acceptance. Naturally, the human psyche attempts to keep track of which therapist is massaging which body part, but the control is eventually surrendered as the massage proceeds.

TASTE

A part of *Ayurveda* that has always intrigued me is the use of a mortar and pestle. What a fun, creative, and magical process. Individualized powdered herbs patiently sit on the shelves, waiting to be mixed together in order to work collectively in the body. Every herb possesses a superior strength that makes it special. It could have more of a digestive capacity, which helps ignite *agni*, or it can have the ability to move into small channels to reach into deeper *dhatus*. Some are heavier to balance *vata dosha*, and some are meant to push *doshas* out in a cleansing manner. Ultimately, when combined in a specific manner, they come together to heal the body.

Loose powders of different colors and aromas are weighed in grams initially. Later, an exact measurement in teaspoons is calculated when given to a patient to take. In India, it was beautiful to see each dose, neatly wrapped in paper, making it easier to take your medicine. There is no such thing as a pill in *Ayurveda*. In fact, we do have tablets, but powder is preferred. Usually, the medicines are given with either ghee, honey, milk, or warm water, and at specific times of the day based on the disease process and *doshas* involved. The patient experiences a true connection with their herbs when the powder form hits the tongue, which is the sense organ related to taste. The sense of taste is awakened and the effect of the herbs are released instantly before even reaching the stomach. There is no need to breakdown a capsule either. The taste of the herbs is generally bitter, but it is fascinating that some individuals actually enjoy the bitterness due to its ability to cool the body down, as it nullifies *pitta dosha* in the internal disease process.

SMELL

Upon entering the clinic, one's sense of smell is immediately awakened, whether from herbs being made to take internally, or a decoction being boiled. If a patient is receiving *panchakarma* (specifically *bastis)*, coarse barks of different herbs are boiled for use in the enemas. This brings the essence of deep-rooted energy into the water to pacify *vata* and move *vata* out of the body. The aroma makes its way into every space of the building, even traveling out into the entrance, masking the smell of garlic from Grimaldi's pizza and connecting us to nature once again.

SOUND

Sounds are present throughout one's journey at the clinic; some externally, some internally, and some through pure noble silence. As any therapeutic session takes place, the chanting helps set the tone in the room. Our own internal chatter also speaks to us as we unwind, unload, and hopefully learn to replace any negative self-defeating thoughts with positive ones. At the right times, the therapists at work are also holding space through noble silence. The *panchakarma* treatments at the clinic require harmony. The *vaman* treatment requires a group of 3-4 therapists. Each therapist performs a different task, whether stroking the patients head, wiping their sweat as it drips, or assisting the patient in the vomiting process. Each therapist works with complete awareness and silence, keeping the patient's needs a priority. We become a family as we take a patient through 7-10 days of an intense process. All of these treatments leave the patient extremely vulnerable and a safe space is held for healing to take place. The survival mechanism in our brain tends to keep our protective defenses in place. As we continue to undergo treatment, we return to a place of sacred vulnerability because we have no choice but *to let go*.

VISION

My vision for every patient I engage with in the therapeutic process is to use my *Ayurvedic Lens* to magnify and uncover the causative factors of my patient's disease process. I hope to guide each patient in the direction of abundance, gifted to us by life and nature.

My vision for the future has been unfolding for the last decade or so. This vision awaits me daily as I work in the clinic that currently stands. A vision dating back to the time I was in naturopathic school. A vision we have as a family. The vision continues to expand into an integrative *center of excellence*. The focus and essence of this center will be to understand and cultivate lifestyles of health and wellness.

CHAPTER NINE

Food As Medicine

Have you ever found yourself wandering around the kitchen, looking for a snack a mere hour after dinner? Or, ever found yourself devouring a piece of cake to satisfy your sweet tooth soon after finishing your lunch? What about eating a bag of potato chips in place of a proper meal? The above scenarios may have been the result of boredom, stress, or perhaps you were simply too busy and unaware of the repercussions. There is a basic understanding that if the previous meal has not been digested fully then it is detrimental to load our *agni* with more. This taxes *agni* and it has to work twice as hard. The effects of this takes years to manifest.

Fundamentals of Digestion

The concept of *agni*, *ama*, and *ojas* are imperative to understanding the digestive process.

Agni—fire, transformation, creation

Agni is known as our transformative power. We have to digest the water we drink, the emotions we experience, and the food we eat. If we fail to do so, *ama* collects, leaving us unsettled.

Ama—sticky, muddy, creates blockages

Ama is any undigested material that shows up in the body, creating symptoms such as sluggishness, pain in the joints, nausea, low appetite, or congestion. It can be easily noticed as a white coating on the tongue first thing in the morning. It is important to scrape the tongue for three main reasons: food tastes better, it prevents halitosis, and it aids in the digestion of food.

Ojas—soft, unctuous, vitality, vigor, strength

The *Samhitas* mention that we are born with eight drops of *ojas* residing in our heart. As we age, those start to get used up. The goal in *Ayurveda* is to seek the best lifestyle to prevent aging. The qualities of *ojas* are best depicted in a newborn baby.

As a society, we are conditioned to view food from the perspective of proteins, carbohydrates, and fat. Even through my naturopathic training in nutrition, we were assessing food in this manner. After becoming immersed in *Ayurveda*, the *gunas* of food are always at the forefront of my mind, enabling me to view food through the lens of how *vata, pitta, kapha* and the seven *dhatus* are affected. To keep it simple, most foods that are white in color and heavy in nature affect *kapha*, foods that are fried, spicy, and fermented affect pitta, and uncooked leafy greens and cold raw foods affect *vata*. To understand how foods affect the *dhatus*, we can take pitta type foods and know that they directly affect *rakta dhatu* due to the relationship between *pitta* and *rakta*. Yogurt and tomatoes are just two examples of foods that can directly vitiate *rakta*.

The beauty of *Ayurveda* lies in the mere fact that every single food, through the six tastes, can be broken down into the five elements. Therefore, the universe becomes our medicinary. In the case of bitter greens, for example, we know that the bitter taste consists of air and space. This air and space equates directly to increasing *vata dosha*, which is made of the same elements.

Six Tastes

The western diet favors sweet, sour, and salty tastes. Before I discovered *Ayurveda*, I also grew up understanding food through these three tastes. I have had my fair share of Cinnamon Toast Crunch cereal, cold milk, cheese, and white bread. It wasn't until I started my *Ayurvedic* studies that I realized that there are three other major taste categories: bitter, pungent, and astringent. It is understood that when all six tastes are present at a meal, we feel balanced and free from cravings, particularly sweet cravings. We often misunderstand the sweet taste, thinking that it only has to do with dessert items. Anything that tastes sweet consists of a substantial amount of earth element. Some examples are wheat, rice, milk, and other grains. Therefore, having any of these items present at our six tastes meal can satisfy the sweet craving.

Food Combining

Smoothies have become extremely popular recently. They are mostly a mixture of cold milk, fruit, ice, yogurt, and possibly some greens. This combination of fruit and milk is not understood by the body. When the body doesn't understand the combination, it is converted into *ama*. The same concept is true for eggs and cheese, a very common breakfast item. Milk and salt, which are the building blocks of cheese, is yet another example. All of these combinations become causative factors for the body which set us up for an array of diseases that settle deep into our tissues.

Ayurvedic Pantry

Spices & Recipes

The following spices and recipes comprise kitchen essentials for a well-stocked *Ayurvedic* pantry. Spices play an important role in *Ayurvedic* daily cooking, as each spice has special qualities which aid in various stages of the digestive process.

Spices

A typical spice box would include: asafoetida, turmeric powder, chili powder, cumin seeds, coriander-cumin powder, mustard seeds, cinnamon sticks, whole cloves, cardamom pods, and salt.

Asafoetida—also known as hing. This spice has an onion-type flavor. Put a dash into your choice of cooking medium (oil or ghee) just 10 seconds before adding your vegetables. It will otherwise burn. Asafoetida is great for dispelling gas. One can mix it with a bit of water and place it on the abdomen like a paste if feeling bloated.

Turmeric powder—mustard yellow in color. It is a root spice, and so, carries with it the energy from the ground. It goes into everything: milk, vegetables, soups, and rice. It is the spice of life. Its strong color is evident in curries. It efficiently cleanses the blood tissue, allowing for healthy *rakta dhatu* formation. It is the anti-everything: antibiotic, anti-inflammatory, antifungal, antiseptic, and anticoagulant. It is used as a paste to cleanse and cool the bride's skin prior to getting married.

Chili powder—pungent in nature. Whole chilis can be dried and put into spicy oil to give flavor or used as a powder.

Cumin seeds—combines well with whole fennel and coriander seeds as a digestive tea. Cooling. Put into oil as it heats up.

Coriander-cumin powder—sweet and grounding. Pair very well together.

Mustard seeds—pungent in nature. Its properties are released when added to heated oil creating a popping sound. Its aroma opens up the channels and has the ability to cleanse negative energy. A few seeds and a small amount of salt can be taken in one hand, circled around the body several times, and thrown away to dispel any negative energy.

Cinnamon sticks—peeled, dried, and rolled bark of a cinnamon tree. Great to use in curries, stews, soups, and rice for extra flavor. Warm, sweet, and pungent in nature.

Whole cloves—aromatic flower buds of a tree. One clove can be added to any dish for added flavor. Even though cloves are hot to taste, they are cooling and soothing for the stomach.

Cardamom pods—light green paper thin pods with small black seeds inside. Often used in Indian sweets and masala chai to give an exotic taste. Sweetly aromatic in nature.

Recipes

—————————— *Kitchari* ——————————

Kitchari is a seasoned mixture of rice and mung dal. Kitchari can be translated to *mixture*. Therefore, you can tailor the ingredients to suit your needs. You can use an array of different vegetables or grains. The mung dal is necessary, though. It is a meal that is capable of nourishing all tissues of the body. Kitchari is rich in protein due to its main ingredient, mung dal. This bean is easy to digest due to the small nature of the bean itself. *Ayurvedically*, kitchari is a *tridoshic* meal, which means that it is suitable for all three constitutions, or *doshic* imbalances: *vata*, *pitta*, and *kapha*. It is also excellent for detoxification and de-aging of the cells. It can be eaten any time an individual wants to give their system a rest.

Ingredients

1 cup mung dal (split yellow or split green or both)

2 cups basmati rice (can also use quinoa or other grains which suit your needs)

8 cups water

1 cinnamon stick

½ teaspoon freshly grated ginger root

3 teaspoons ghee

½ teaspoon turmeric powder

½ teaspoon coriander-cumin powder

½ teaspoon cumin seeds

½ teaspoon mustard seeds

¼ teaspoon salt

A dash of asafoetida (hing)

Handful of fresh cilantro leaves finely chopped

1½ cups assorted fresh vegetables—zucchini, carrots, sweet potato, corn, peas, and onions can be used.

Preparation

- Carefully pick over rice and dal to remove any stones or impurities. Wash in at least two changes of water. If time allows, let the mung dal soak for a few hours before cooking, as it helps with digestibility. If you have a particularly difficult time digesting beans, you may want to precook the beans for 20-30 minutes using 4 cups of water.

- Warm 1-2 teaspoons of ghee in a saucepan or pressure cooker. Add mustard and cumin seeds. Add a dash of asafoetida once the seeds pop. You may add chopped onions and let them brown a bit. Add the rice, mung dal mixture, and fresh vegetables. Add some water. Season with turmeric, fresh ginger, cumin coriander powder, a cinnamon stick, salt, and stir.

- Add another 2 teaspoons of ghee and add enough water to cover all contents in the saucepan or pressure cooker. Bring to a boil for 5 minutes, uncovered, stirring occasionally. Turn down the heat to low and cover, leaving the lid slightly ajar. Cook until tender, about 20-25 minutes. If using a pressure cooker wait for 3 whistles.

- Garnish with fresh cilantro and serve. Serves 6.

Mung Dal Soup

Ingredients

2 cups split green mung dal (can also add a combination of whole green mung dal soaked overnight and green split or even yellow mung dal split on its own)

8 cups water

A dash of asafoetida (hing)

1 star of anise (optional)

2 tablespoons ghee / olive oil

1 ¼ teaspoon turmeric powder

1 teaspoon cumin seeds

1 teaspoon salt

1 whole clove

¼ teaspoon chili powder

2 teaspoons freshly grated ginger root

2 teaspoons mustard seeds (less for *pitta*, more for *vata* and *kapha*)

1 teaspoon coriander-cumin powder

½ onion, chopped

1 garlic clove, chopped

1 green chili (optional)

Fresh lemon

Handful of fresh cilantro leaves finely chopped

Preparation

- Wash dal until water runs clear. If using whole mung beans, soak the night before and leave on the counter top. No need to soak if they are split. Grate ginger and chop vegetables beforehand.
- You may cook the mung dal in a pressure cooker or in a saucepan.
- Warm 2 tablespoons of ghee/oil in a large, heavy saucepan or pressure cooker. Once ghee heats up, add mustard seeds, cumin seeds, and a dash of asafoetida to the ghee. May need to turn the heat down so the ghee doesn't burn. If you would like, you may sauté onions, garlic, green chili, and ginger in the oil/ghee for flavor.
- Add mung beans in any variation. Cover with enough water for a soupy consistency. Then, season with cumin-coriander powder, turmeric, chili, clove, and salt. Reduce to low-medium heat to cook. If the beans weren't soaked prior to cooking, cook time may increase. If using a pressure cooker 3 whistles will suffice.
- Garnish soup with fresh cilantro and lemon. Serves 4-6

Spicy Oil

There is a particular order to the addition of spices while cooking. The purpose of the spices is to add flavor, aid in digestion, and satisfy all six tastes.

Ingredients

2 tablespoons ghee or any cooking medium

1 teaspoon mustard seeds

1 teaspoon cumin seeds

½ teaspoon turmeric powder

¼ - ½ teaspoon chili powder

½ teaspoon coriander-cumin powder

2 teaspoons freshly grated ginger root

A dash of asafoetida (hing)

Salt as required

1 clove garlic, chopped

½ onion, chopped

1 green chili (optional)

1 tablespoon fresh cilantro leaves finely chopped

Fresh lemon

Preparation

- Heat oil (any medium including ghee, olive oil, or coconut oil) in a skillet. As soon as the oil heats up, add mustard seeds. When they begin to pop, add cumin seeds and a dash of asafoetida.

- Only allow 10 seconds for the asafoetida to be in the oil because it will burn. Add onions, garlic, and green chilis as needed.

- Add other vegetables, dal, rice, or a combination of these.

- Spice up the mixture with the addition of cumin-coriander powder (usually comes already mixed as one), chili powder, turmeric, and salt.

- After cooking is complete, garnish with lemon and cilantro.

Ghee

Ghee is used widely in Indian and *Ayurvedic* cooking. It can be used on a daily basis while cooking and can also be used as a base for many herbal remedies. One can make their own medicated gold ghee by allowing a piece of real gold jewelry (at least five to ten grams) to circulate in the ghee while boiling. The effects of gold are numerous. It can help to nullify negativity in the body of any kind—emotional, physical, and mental. Ghee has the ability to increase *ojas*, enhance *agni*, internally lubricate the tissues, and cool the body by balancing *pitta*. Unsalted butter is typically used.

Ingredients

2 sticks (1 cup) unsalted butter (or as much as you want to make)

Preparation

- Use a medium sized, heavy bottom saucepan. Make sure it is dry and clean. Place the butter in the pan and cook uncovered on medium heat until all the butter melts.
- Continue cooking, stirring occasionally, until the butter starts to foam and boil. You will hear crackling; this means the butter is boiling.
- Reduce heat to low and continue to simmer the butter until it clarifies—when you part the foam on top, you should see the melted butter getting clearer.

- Continue to simmer the butter until the crackling subsides, about 10 minutes. How soon the ghee is done will vary depending on the quantity of butter you are using, so reference the indicators below.

The ghee is done when:

- The crackling subsides. This means most of the moisture has been cooked away.
- The liquid becomes clear golden yellow color in color (part the foam with a spoon to see the ghee).
- The milk solids separate and settle in the bottom of the pan, and are light brown in color. Be careful not to overcook the ghee and burn the solids. If the milk solids are dark brown, or if the liquid ghee turns dark brown, you've over cooked it.

Other facts:

- Let the ghee cool for about 20 minutes. Then strain it though a very fine strainer or two layers of muslin cloth. Make sure all the milk solids are strained out; strain the ghee twice if needed.
- Store ghee in a clean, dry bottle. Do not put a lid on the container until the ghee is fully cooled.
- Ghee can be stored at room temperature; no need for refrigeration.

Ayurvedic Spiced Milk

Milk is considered a *rasayana* in *Ayurveda*. Therefore, it has the capability of deeply nourishing and replenishing our tissues. Adding the following spices to the milk as well as allowing the milk to come to a boil allows for easy digestion in those who normally feel they have a tough time digesting milk. This spiced milk is great just before bed if you are having trouble falling or staying asleep. Wonderful for kids as well.

Ingredients

> 1 cup organic cow's milk
>
> Pinch of cardamom powder or 1 whole pod
>
> Pinch of nutmeg
>
> Pinch of turmeric powder
>
> 1 strand saffron
>
> 1 teaspoon ghee
>
> 1 teaspoon sugar

Preparation

- Pour milk (preferably organic) in a saucepan.
- Add nutmeg, turmeric, cardamom, saffron, ghee (if desired), and sugar.
- Bring the milk to a boil once or twice.
- No need to strain. Simply drink and enjoy. Serves 1.

Masala Chai

Ingredients

1 cup organic cow's milk

1 cup water

1 black tea bag or 1 teaspoon loose black tea leaves

1 teaspoon sugar (adjust to your liking)

¼ teaspoon freshly grated ginger root

⅛ teaspoon cardamom powder or 2 whole cardamom pods

*Ready-made tea masala powder can be purchased (usually a mixture of dry ginger, cardamom, cinnamon and nutmeg). Can also make this at home on your own.

Preparation

- Bring black tea and water to a boil.
- As ingredients are boiling add freshly grated ginger, tea masala (can buy this ready-made), cardamom, and sugar.
- When water and ingredients come to a boil, add milk and bring to a boil once or twice more.
- Strain and drink. The ratio is about 1 cup water to 1 cup milk. If making more, adjust accordingly. Serves 1

CHAPTER TEN

An Attitude Of Gratitude
While Traveling

Traveling can be transformative. All of our senses are engaged in the journey. Breathing the air, visualizing new colors, hearing the language, smelling authentic foods, and taking in the landscape makes each journey special.

Splendor of India

Vivid memories surface of our travels throughout India. The vibrant colors used in embroidered pieces, the traditional garb of the village people, and the food stalls on the side of a rickety road are just a few images I keep close. I remember stopping at a small restaurant on the side of the street on our way to Bhuj. There was nothing else in sight. We sat down, and I wondered if they were really going to give us something to eat? We ordered and our bill came to 50 cents a person. What a bargain! How could such great food be only 50 cents?

After a long day of travel, we arrived in Bhuj. Picture this: all of the rooms were situated, overlooking the lobby. The person taking care of the hotel would pull his cot out and retire for the night in the open space below. In order to shower, we had to fill buckets with water from across the hall. He told us to come for dinner. He led us up to a place on the rooftop. He started placing these small *bhakris* (semolina bread) on our plates. I couldn't believe how my taste buds were reacting. I could feel the love that these *bhakris* started to add to my being. They were delicious as they were dipped in ghee—warm butter in its most pure golden form. This beautiful experience remains imprinted upon my psyche.

That same trip, we traveled into a village where we watched traditional Indian fabrics being woven on a loom. The women were working so hard, but they had such joy on their faces. At that time, we were on the lookout for unique wedding favors. We had the idea of asking the villagers to make *dandiyas*, which are wooden sticks used in traditional dancing as part of Indian wedding festivities. The guests could take them home as wedding favors. Completely non-toxic color was used to design these wooden sticks. We also had the villagers make some of our outfits. We were shocked at the ease with which all of this was shipped back to the United States.

Later, we managed to catch a glimpse of a process known as block printing. The patterns being printed on the scarves were beautiful. All the materials were completely natural. My mom must have bought 20 of them.

These experiences happened about eight years ago. These encounters have shaped my being deeper than I can intellectualize. Traveling has a way of transporting us through air and space to something outside of us. Something deeper that has a way of opening up our hearts and minds. I have developed a tremendous amount of gratitude from my trip to this remote part of India.

The Incan Trail

In 2011, we undertook a family trip to Machu Picchu. A 40-mile trek lay ahead of us. We were all challenged consistently beyond our comfort zone. My husband and I lagged behind the rest of the group. How could it be any other way? My mom and sisters trekked ahead at the front. It was a time to be strong, to realize our true colors, and observe both our internal nature as well as the natural world around us. I wished that we could have all stayed together. We just had to feel what it was like and accept our differences in body type. What were we going to do? Mother Nature was teaching us to trust our bodies. I doubted my ability to complete the trek. We had a few practice sessions with some smaller treks beforehand, not to mention extreme conditioning on the stair master.

I started feeling very dizzy the night before the trek. They had to give me oxygen in our room. I was also prescribed a diuretic. I was suffering from an intense headache as well. I struggled taking the pharmaceuticals, but I had to if I wanted to join the rest of my family on the trek. I had packed an *Ayurvedic* first aid kit, but I was not in the position to even try that. I needed instant relief. This was a time when I had to surrender. I was determined. My breathing had become so shallow. They say those over 30 years of age have a tougher time with altitude changes, but somehow I managed. I took it easy. As long as I was taking the diuretic, I was okay.

There was a moment that will always remain outlined in my head. My husband and I were traversing the most challenging part of the hike. It was around this time that we started to give up and drag a bit. Magically, our amazing porters showed up. Imagine, the porters were shoeless. Ironically, as we prepared for the trek, we focused on buying the best shoes possible with the best tread. The porters sped right past us, some completely barefoot and some with humble flip-flops. The porters took both of our backpacks in order to lessen our load. With their help, we made it. The food, tents, and breathtaking views awaited us. Gratitude for such a travel experience comes to mind. We must thank Mother Earth for providing the opportunity to experience challenges with nature's sounds, sights, and smells.

What is gratitude? Gratitude is the *quality* of being thankful and appreciative. I honestly cannot say I knew the meaning for myself until my global travels. It is a state of mind that we constantly, actively cultivate. Our waking thoughts of gratitude are received and magnified by the universe.

CHAPTER ELEVEN

Collective Female Consciousness

O ur core group of women thus far includes my mom, my two younger sisters, my daughter Veda, and I. My Indian culture, loving family ties, and desire for harmony is empowering. I believe women have a special place in this world. I have thought about this repeatedly and consider the beauty of our collective female energy a privilege that only appears with consistent internal work and a highly dedicated mother. This familial bonding didn't happen overnight. I consider my mom the glue that keeps us together. Without her, we would all fall apart. She is the perfect example of an inspirational figure with qualities we should all aspire to express. The three of us, having come from a single parent family and having overcome numerous hurdles, have developed the tools to persevere. *Ayurveda* is at the core of our beings. We all understand the principles and abide by them. Family should be able to follow similar principles in order to ride the same wave. Through our journeys such as traveling, meditating, and simply being together, we have been able to communicate deeply and be our true selves.

My mom is like a lioness leading her pack. She was born and raised in East Africa. She has shared many of life's lessons with us. She is a psychiatrist, teacher, writer, yogini, meditator, and ultimately, a strong, loving ball of enlightenment. She is a true testament to her *pitta prakruti*. She doesn't waver. Steadfast, she maintains healthy habits, including meditation, *abhyanga* oil massage, and yearly *panchakarmas*. She shows the same dedication in her work as a physician, her vision, and most of all, her gifts as a mother. We learn from her and aspire to be like her. She has enriched our lives deeply. I truly love her and have a profound connection to her. Actually, it is written in the stars. In Vedic astrology, my chart depicts the mother in the fourth house. No wonder I ended up staying here in Arizona, allowing us to keep our strong bond, a lesson in how life decisions can make such an impact.

She consistently knows how to manage conflict and is always teaching us to process our emotions. I have seen her at work during a few patients' psychotherapy sessions; she is brilliant in deciphering an individual's life path. I will always remember her words: *Psychotherapy helps us understand, while a spiritual practice is crucial to letting go.* An *Ayurvedic* lifestyle along with yearly *panchakarma* has been extremely helpful. She is in awe when any one *Ayurvedic* herb produces great results. She exclaims, "What was that? It was magical. It saved me." She is dedicated to life, love, and overcoming barriers to her well-being. Strength on all levels is my mantra for her.

I have a special relationship with each sister. The youngest, Meera, is a beautiful soul. I started to get to know her on a deeper level during a trip to Seattle when I was 18. She is seven years younger than me. She has completed medical school and is on her way to training as an integrative psychiatrist. She is a wise being, and I attribute it to her starting to meditate at a very young age. Her *prakruti* resides in *vata*. She has always been extremely creative, so much so that she has the last say in our collective art projects. Always having complained of being the youngest, she is now relieved of that burden, as Veda, her niece, has assumed that role.

Pooja, my middle sister, is another beautiful soul. She has been gifted the art of making people feel and look beautiful through her artistic abilities. She is a true act of *pitta* ready to take over the world, making her way into the fashion and beauty industry with determination.

Veda, my 14-month-old daughter, is a ball of happiness who aches to explore the world and venture into every nook and cranny. She lights up all of our lives and is a shining beam of light through which we can see the world. Being around her is likely to dissipate any aches, pains, or worries. How can a little ball of light magnify our lives? She is godlike, full of purity, love, harmony, and sweetness.

We are a soul cluster. We are powerful, both together and as individuals. This is what collective energy can do. This is how relationships are meant to develop. We have to do our best to be full within ourselves in order to manage our relationships and evolve on a common path. We are all on the same path, we just come in at different points.

CHAPTER TWELVE

Silencing The Monkey Mind

A universal meditation technique known as *Vipassana* was first accessible to me at the age of 18. My grandparents were assistant teachers to the late *Goenka-ji* who carried this technique in its pristine form from Burma. They taught all over Europe before they immigrated to the United States. I sat my first three-day sit as a teenager in Shelburne Falls, Massachusetts. Soon after, I began to participate in ten-day noble silence retreats. I attended my first sit with my mother. After that, I sat with my husband (prior to our marriage), a dear friend, and with family several times. My most recent noble silence retreat was when I was five months pregnant with my daughter.

These ten-day silent retreats are structured around silence, and through maintaining this silence, we naturally begin to journey inward and become aware of our mental impurities. The term *Vipassana* literally translates into *seeing things as they really are.* It is a true testament of what it's like to be with ourselves. After all, we are alone in this world and we are ultimately responsible for our emotions and whatever misery may lie inside. We are constantly looking for happiness outside of ourselves. Each course has increased my awareness and created more space for me to fall deeper in love with my being.

I remember my first ten-day sit vividly. I suffered from splitting headaches almost daily. Now, looking back through an *Ayurvedic Lens*, I realized that I failed to understand that these hot, sharp sensations with an irritating nature must have been a collection of *pitta* energy rising to the surface, seeking escape. It is not important to know why or what contributed to this *dosha* accumulation, but once again, to understand that everything boils down to the elements in the body that don't serve us. The signs are there when we begin to fall out of balance. Being present and observing these signs allow us to catch them when they are still young, weak, and influential. When we let these early signs pass us by, disease starts to set in and the *doshas* begin to find a home in our tissues.

The course that my husband and I sat through together was a great way to strengthen our bond and clear any blockages before getting married. Ironically enough, it was a bond strengthened through noble silence. My grandmother had always advised us to sit together before getting married. It is a wonderful test of your ability to be *within* in the presence of your partner. It made me realize that we are in this life to observe our nature. By doing so, we unburden our own being and create space that enables us to develop greater intimacy in our relationships. Both people in a relationship must work towards evolving in order to sustain the challenges life brings forth. Your true *prakruti* awaits you every step of the way.

I was five months pregnant at my most recent ten-day course. The fifth month is significant because the baby's senses are awakened, open, and ready to receive. This little *dhamma* baby was absorbing the Buddhist teachings taught in one of the oldest languages, *Pali*. This experience has helped shape her consciousness and has allowed her to start collecting *parmis* (Buddha-like qualities) at a young age. The teachers always told me to observe her body language and her behavior compared to other kids her age. My youngest sister recently sat a course and it dawned on her that Veda's first word was *appy*. An interesting coincidence, as it is so close phonetically to *happy*. Anyone who sees her instantly feels the happiness that exudes from her being. She is a treat and I am grateful for all the guidance that I received to create a positive experience in the natural birthing process.

Vipassana meditation has been an anchor to my being. The principles of *Vipassana* have penetrated into each of my cells, bringing intelligence at the right moments: during the birth of my daughter, when making difficult decisions, and when communicating with compassion. Sitting these retreats has kept all of our relationships strong by creating deep love for each other. My grandparents searched high and low to bring the greatness of such a path into our lives.

I still remember how dedicated my grandmother was to this technique. *Ba* was what we called her. She came to live in

Scottsdale just before she passed. Looking back, she exuded a *pitta prakruti* with exceptional organizational skills. She was worldly, practical, logical, an amazing cook, had a good sense of humor, and always loved from a place of warmth in her heart. She was so faithful to this *Vipassana* technique, and I can think of no better story to illustrate this than the following: During my naturopathic training she lived with my sister and I in a beautiful home in north Scottsdale. She had her own living quarters tucked away toward the east end of the home. There were days when I would come home from school and make my way to her room. The door would be closed, and there would be a sign on the door which read: *One-day sit in progress; observing noble silence, food is on the stove.* She was a true testament of beauty—dedicated to herself and yet able to take care of other's needs. I can hardly imagine what went on in her room, with her closely following the meditation timetable and setting up a space in her room to meditate. She would venture out occasionally, still in noble silence, when breaks were allowed.

My grandfather was just as rooted in his being. *Dadaji* was what we called him. He was a man of few words. I remember a specific conversation I had with him about his self-led study of homeopathy. We chatted for an hour or so one evening about his discovery. This science fascinated him. Homeopathy is described as a vibrational medicine in which likes and dislikes related to diet and lifestyle are uncovered. Questions about what makes a disease process or a set of symptoms better or worse are also asked. We worked through a couple of cases together. He would study this science on his own time, as his true profession was that of a surgeon. My mom tells me he was well-versed in the readings of the *Bhagavad Gita*. His aim after reading this was how he could best incorporate the principles of the *Bhagavad Gita* into action. He tried many different meditation techniques before landing on *Vipassana*. He was searching for guidance of how to live life on a mental, emotional, and spiritual level.

My grandparents were appointed as teachers to the late *Goenka-Ji*. Both of them have now passed and after such extraordinary lives! Growing up in East Africa, becoming physicians, and escaping the exodus to find enlightenment are just a few examples of the extraordinary stations they passed through in their lives. They would be happy to know that we have all adopted this technique and even their great granddaughter has received Buddha's teachings in utero. My mom repeatedly says *if only we had these tools when we were your age.*

There are ten *parmis*, or, qualities of Buddha-hood that one can begin to master after having sat a course. I see the qualities that both my grandmother and grandfather have passed on into our family through their experience. My grandmother always showed strong determination through all of her efforts; in *Pali* the word is *addhitana*. My grandfather showed great perseverance in locating the best meditation technique possible.

These courses are strictly donation based and therefore create the opportunity to be able to serve at retreats. Serving at retreats is the best way to give back to those who have served you.

Ayurveda teaches us to allow *manas*, our mind, to remain as *sattvic* as possible. Through meditation of any kind, we can strengthen our mind and not allow the three *doshas* to accumulate. Meditation serves to not only increase our *sattvic* nature, but also balance *vata* that is out of control. *Goenka-ji* constantly refers to our monkey mind, grabbing hold of anything and everything that comes in our path. We rarely step back, widening our lens in order to realize that we are reacting to outside forces and, furthermore, blaming our miseries on factors that lie outside of us. We must tame our monkey mind and find equanimity. Equanimity, in *Pali* called *upekha*, refers to the ability to maintain balance of the mind through challenging experiences. This *parmi* resonates strongly with my being. I am always striving to live life from this place.

Prana translates into life force. *Prana* runs through *rakta*, our blood tissue, giving us *jiva* (life). If our breathing is shallow, too fast, or absent, our life force becomes depleted. From the first to the last, our breathing continues. I've witnessed both—I've now seen my daughter take her first breath, as well as my grandfather take his last. Veda's introduction to the world was accompanied by crying, while my grandfather's passing occurred with great ease. One would expect quite the opposite—that we would die with great misery—but in his case, through his practice of *Vipassana*, he took his last breaths with a smile on his face. He showed me the art of dying, as he used all the principles of *Vipassana* through his last hours, minutes, and seconds with us.

Reference for Vipassana: www.dhamma.org

CHAPTER THIRTEEN

A Look Through
Your *Ayurvedic Lens*

How did *Ayurveda* literally save my life? I was headed down the wrong path, and I don't think any other healing modality could have brought me back to where I am today. *Ayurveda* saved Veda's life as well, as it is understood that health is passed down through each subsequent generation. Without my dedicated family members, who have entertained the idea of yearly cleansing and have had constant faith as I guided them through their health journeys, I would not have had the experiences that shape my being. I have deep gratitude for my stellar patients for their continued trust, which has rewarded them with deep knowledge at a cellular level. Deep in my heart rests my love for my gurus, all of whom continue to travel with me in spirit as I perform each examination, herbal preparation, or *panchakarma* process.

What is it that continually draws us back to this ancient wisdom? Dr. Deepak Chopra is largely responsible for thrusting *Ayurveda* into mainstream consciousness. *Ayurveda* is gaining momentum, just as yoga has. We should make every effort to continue to raise awareness about *Ayurveda*.

Habits are harder to change as we age. We can see the effects of the changes we make most readily in future generations.

The science of yoga took time to become popular, but now there is a yoga studio on every street corner. After all, *Ayurveda* is the sister science of yoga. The term *popular* is used here to refer to fads that have gained traction such as vegan, raw, paleo, gluten-free, juicing, and dairy-free. We are robbing ourselves of the very nutrition that started our evolution. Such questions abound in our modern world, as should we have high protein meals, fermented foods or be vegetarian? These queries have only come forth because we have lost touch with ourselves, venturing far away from our roots. We tend to blame it on the times, stress, and too much external stimuli. It is important to take responsibility for your health by exploring what feels right rather than blindly following because it's the new fad or a new study that just came out. It takes magnifying, focusing, and zooming in with commitment and responsibility.

Ayurvedic medicine has a way of healing our beings. Patients who have tried everything become the best patients. They are finally able to trust and surrender to ancient wisdom, no longer brainwashed by the principles of modern medicine. Current medical practice emphasizes looking externally for answers, popping pills, and treating each system separately. The voice that screams out *Heal me, please!* predominates, igniting the desire for personal responsibility in healing. This inner voice speaks up, saying: *Use your Ayurvedic Lens to assess me and I promise, I too will use my Ayurvedic Lens to dig deeper inside and journey within. I will no longer escape. I will take responsibility for whatever traumas have occurred. I will stop resisting now that I have identified my triggers, and I will keep the door wide open. I will stop being a victim of my past. I will venture into the present. Although it hurts to uncover the truth, I know it is worth the pain.*

I live, eat, and breathe *Ayurveda* daily. In this vast *vata* vitiated world, we managed to find each other and become entangled with no chance of separation. There was a point where I had veered off my path, having forgotten my roots, my core being, and what I was capable of becoming. *Ayurveda* has been my guiding force, giving me the deepest answers to these questions and allowing me to unpeel those layers necessary to rediscover my true being. This journey has given me the tools to be an effective and authentic mentor for others. Daily, my eyes align with *The Ayurvedic Lens*. I use it to zoom further into understanding disease, *doshas*, relationships, and life at its best.

I have arisen from my roots only to continue on this path moment by moment using all the tools I have collected along the way. I invite you to join your being on this journey, as you begin to observe life through your own *Ayurvedic Lens*, allowing you to reap the benefits of a cleanse, build strong wholesome relationships with yourself and others, parent with compassion, meditate to settle the monkey mind, give birth naturally, exercise with the intention of digesting our *doshas* rather than losing weight, and explore your *Ayurvedic* pantry of herbs, spices, and recipes to pacify your *doshic* imbalances.

Glossary

Abhyanga: oil massage

Agni: digestive fire

Ahara: diet or food

Ama: any undigested material that cannot be utilized by the body

Amrita: pot containing rejuvenating nectar

Asana: yoga pose

Asthi: bone

Avayava: organ

Ayur: life or longevity

Ayurveda: science of life

Basti: one of five panchakarma therapies using either oil or decoction based enemas to remove vitiated vata dosha

Bramacharya: balanced sexual drive

Charaka: Ayurvedic author

Chinta: mental activity, especially thinking

Dhanvantari: personal physician to the Divine beings

Dhatu: one of the body's seven components; tissue

Dosha: three energies believed to circulate in the body and govern physical activity

Guna: tendency, quality, or attribute

Hetu: causative factor

Hruday: heart

Jalouka: leeches

Jiva: individual soul; life

Kapha: one of three doshas comprised of predominantly water and earth elements governing the structure of the body

Karana: cause

Karma: action

Karya: effect

Mahabutas: five elements including space, air, fire, water, and earth

Majja: bone marrow, nerve tissue

Manas: mind

Mansa: muscle

Marma: vital points on the body

Meda: fat

Nasya: one of five panchakarma therapies involving the administration of nasal medications

Nidra:	sleep
Ojas:	pure and subtle substance that is extracted from food that has been completely digested; vigor
Panchakarma:	five cleansing/detoxification actions involving vomiting, purgation, enemas, bloodletting, and nasal medications to remove doshas from the body
Pitta:	one of three doshas comprised of predominantly fire and water elements governing transformation in the body
Prakruti:	an individual's distinctive constitution
Prana:	life force
Rajas:	one of three gunas characterized by activity, stimulation, and movement
Rakta:	blood
Raktamokshan:	one of five panchakarma therapies involving bloodletting either with leeches or needles to remove vitiated rakta and pitta
Rasa:	plasma
Rasayana:	Any herb, food, or activity which promotes youthfulness and cures disease

Samhita: any methodically arranged collection of texts or verses

Sattva: the purest of the three gunas characterized by equilibrium and intelligence

Shankh: conch shell

Shukra: reproductive fluid

Shushruta: Ayurvedic author

Sneha: oil or any unctuous substance

Srotas: channels of circulation in the body

Sudarshan Chakra: spinning disc-like weapon

Tamas: one of the three gunas characterized by inertia

Vaghbhata: Ayurvedic author

Vaman: one of five panchakarma therapies involving medicated emesis which removes vitiated kapha dosha

Vata: one of three doshas comprised of predominantly air and space elements governing movement in the body

Veda: knowledge

Vikruti: a disordered physical constitution resulting from an imbalance of doshas

Virechan: one of five panchakarma therapies involving purgation which removes vitiated pitta dosha

About the Book

This book is a compilation of stories, patient cases, educational material, and an account of close personal relationships viewed through the lens of the world's oldest system of healing—*Ayurveda*. *Ayur* means life, and *Veda* means science. Together, these translate into the *science of life*. It is through the principles of *Ayurveda*, that one can begin to understand how we function, how we show up in the world, and what makes us tick.

This book is meant to touch those who feel burdened, stuck, or ill and would like to clear their path. It is meant to help those who strive to feel lighter, happier, joyful... *more alive*. It's also for those who are tired of trying to figure it out on their own. It is a recipe book for living life in abundance.

This recipe book for life has a variety of ingredients: Its mainstay is *Ayurvedic* medicine with all of its lifestyle components (i.e. meditation, cooking, oil massage, exercise, pre and post partum care, detoxification, and journaling). This manuscript consists of the purest path in life I know of thus far. It will show you all the cards in the deck, the ace card being how to live a healthier, longer life. You will learn the best coping skills to help you through every stage of your life.

It will help you dig into your roots, find out more about yourself, and explore your desires, your mysteries, and your story.

You will enter into a creative journey with yourself using the science of *Ayurveda* as your guide. This ancient wisdom

146 Dr. Meghana Thanki, NMD

is awaiting your presence, and it will stand by you from the toughest of times to the happiest of times and everything in between, as you peer through your *Ayurvedic Lens* in journeying into your desire to heal.

About the Author

Dr. Thanki is a Naturopathic Physician specializing in *Ayurvedic* medicine. She is a wife, mother, physician, yoga teacher, *Vipassana* meditator, writer, and traveler. Her practice is located in sunny Scottsdale, Arizona. Dr. Thanki eats, breathes, and lives in the authenticity of *Ayurvedic* medicine. It penetrates her being every moment, as that is how she views the world and nature daily; through an *Ayurvedic Lens*. She brings her deep understanding of *Ayurvedic* principles to patients as she shepherds them through the process of *panchakarma* detoxification, assists in making the connection between *Ayurvedic* food as medicine, and discusses with her patients how to make more positive lifestyle changes to complete the journey inward.

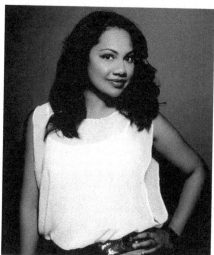

Photo credit © Michael Franco

Patient Testimonials

"Health is Happiness *Ayurveda* and Dr. Thanki have brought my Health and Happiness back!"

"I am amazed by the incredible power of natural healing through *Ayurveda*. Having come to you initially with some very serious addictions, I am pleased at the progress we have made in transforming my lifestyle. I have been drug and smoke free for over a year now and have every reason to believe these are life-long changes. You have given me invaluable tools and guiding principles that have been instrumental in creating a new way of life that is nourishing and sustaining. For so many years I was looking for something outside of myself to give me what I have had within me all along. We have come a long way, but I also feel like this is just the beginning, and I look forward to the many years to come, including a continuation of your guidance and wisdom."

"Panchakarma with Dr. Thanki was one of the best things I have done for myself. I would recommend that everyone try this at least once. I felt rejuvenated and energized as well as had an increased clarity of mind. I'm very thankful for having had the privilege of working with Dr. Meghana Thanki and her phenomenal expertise and treatments. I would recommend her to anyone."